Digital Dental Implantology

Jorge M. Galante • Nicolás A. Rubio

Editors

Digital Dental Implantology

From Treatment Planning to Guided Surgery

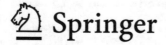

Springer

Editors
Jorge M. Galante
Universidad de Buenos Aires
Ciudad Autónoma de Buenos Aires
Argentina

Nicolás A. Rubio
Universidad de Buenos Aires
Ciudad Autónoma de Buenos Aires
Argentina

ISBN 978-3-030-65949-3   ISBN 978-3-030-65947-9   (eBook)
https://doi.org/10.1007/978-3-030-65947-9

This Springer imprint is published by the registered company Springer Nature Switzerland AG
The registered company address is: Gewerbestrasse 11, 6330 Cham, Switzerland

Prologue

Fusing CBCT and CAD/CAM technologies seems to be the right path to follow if wanting to improve accuracy and predictability in surgical dental treatments. Another great advantage about using a digital approach is time reduction in surgical procedures, thus decreasing patient morbidity significantly.

On one hand, CBCT is one of the most helpful diagnostic tools available nowadays and has become mandatory whenever indicating implant therapy. This new tomography system has evolved to give detailed information about tissue topography while reducing radiation exposure time for the benefit of the patient. Its usefulness in surgical diagnosis is far beyond questionable. Usually, CBCT images are presented in printed paper and slices are defined by the professional in charge of performing the study. Nevertheless, slices can always be customized, segmentations can be done, and other parameters can be managed to obtain specific information. For that means, an image processing software is needed.

On the other hand, a new era has recently begun, where physical objects can be digitalized in order to manipulate them, make modifications or even create a new object based on the original. To accomplish that, every object has to be scanned and turned into a digital surface image. Again, this process requires a specific software.

To resume, two different technologies are available in dental daily practice: CBCT and digital casts. Many advantages come from fusing the digitalized "external surface" of an object (i.e., dental arch) with the digital image of the object "inner aspect" (i.e., maxillary tomography). This book explains the merging process involved, its advantages, and its applications in oral surgery.

The first step to begin understanding the fusing process is to highlight the need of two different digital files, DICOM and STL files. These are two different languages to express a digital file, like .doc and .pdf files. To simplify, DICOM files are created from CBCT equipments, while STL files are created from scanners. A combined image can be obtained by merging both files using a software. Tooth anatomy is usually used as reference point to put images together, as its surface is registered both by the CBCT and the scan. Merging process is the most critical step of the whole virtual planning. Accuracy is essential at this point to assure predictability. Patients prostheses or templates are also used in cases where tooth anatomy is partially or totally absent.

The second step is to determine your treatment plan. For that means, digital wax up can be used to stablish a prosthetically driven surgery, if not been done previously. Prosthodontic plan leads to surgical plan and so, the software allows to perform virtual surgery practice. If implant placement is the main objective, virtual implants are placed; if bone regeneration needs to be addressed, virtual implants are placed and bone is virtually shaped to contain said implants.

The third step is template manufacturing. In other words, once surgical project is reviewed and accepted, accurate template must be fabricated to reproduce virtual planning. Even though this process is done fluidly, careful assessment during template construction is necessary to obtain a perfect fit. Materials used to fabricate surgical guides vary according to the surgical protocol.

The digital approach proposed in this book stablishes a paradigm shift. Despite general belief, this approach demands a lot of time, hard work, and a rather slow learning curve to get the best out of it. Moreover, guided surgery protocols stand for exhaustive diagnosis and increasing time spent on the virtual phase in order to decrease chair-side time. Thus, the aim of guided surgery philosophy is to improve diagnosis, be able to reproduce the planning and reduce patient morbidity. This book serves as a guide to initiate clinicians in the exciting world of technology fusion and to understand the advantages and limitations of the digital approach.

Jorge M. Galante
Universidad de Buenos Aires
Ciudad Autónoma de Buenos Aires
Argentina

Nicolás A. Rubio
Universidad de Buenos Aires
Ciudad Autónoma de Buenos Aires
Argentina

Contents

Part I

Digital Workflow in Dental Surgery

1.1 CAI/CAD/CAM Concept

Nicolás A. Rubio

The dental digital workflow can be divided into three global steps, regardless the process involved; either for surgical, prosthodontic or orthodontic use. Each step has to be carefully addressed in order to achieve a precise outcome. Errors in the initial phase can lead to serious mistakes, despite meticulous treatment planning. Said steps in the digital workflow refer to:

– Computer-Assisted Imaging (CAI): It is the initial step of the process and stands for digital data acquisition. Although often disregarded, this stage is critical to ensure a reliable result. While digital planning seems to be easy-going, no software will indicate if the uploaded data is erroneous, altered or does not match patient clinical situation. Therefore, special considerations have to be taken into account for the optimization of the image capturing procedure.
– Computer-Assisted Design (CAD): It represents the surgical virtual planning stage and uses a dental software. A huge variety of these computer programs can be found, from license restricted to license free; from simply image viewers to advanced planning software. They serve as great tools for diagnosis and treatment planning and additionally, allow to export data to help accomplish the desired outcome. The designing phase demands expertise and therefore, a time-consuming training.
– Computer-Assisted Manufacturing (CAM): To translate the virtual plan to the analog and tangible scenario, a device needs to be manufactured. Moreover, ad hoc tools, such as specific surgical drills, are necessary during the clinical procedure. Also, a special software is needed to control the machines in charge of the manufacturing process. This step is usually trusted to the dental technician, as it implies additional equipment.

To summarize, the first important step is to acquire digital data from patient anatomy while minimizing volume alterations and maximizing surface definition (CAI). Next, the information is uploaded into a dental software where the virtual surgery is performed and the whole planning is confirmed (CAM). Afterwards, data is exported to a machine which creates a physical object to be used prior or during surgery (CAD).

It is important to outline that the clinician can interact and participate actively in every phase or trust some steps to a third party. Nevertheless, knowledge of the whole process is mandatory to ensure a predictable outcome.

CAI: Computer-Assisted Imaging

Nicolás A. Rubio

1.1 Introduction

Acquiring reliable digital data from the patient is fundamental for accomplishing a correct diagnosis and a trustworthy treatment plan. For that means, clinicians need to obtain 2 types of data: surface scans from patient oral cavity and medical images from the underlying tissue anatomy.

On one side, knowledge of bone anatomy and tissue thickness is undoubtedly necessary when planning surgery. Thus, medical instruments have evolved to provide neat and detailed images, which can be displayed in any computer in order to achieve a precise diagnosis. Therefore, a universal medical language has been stablished to visualize these images: the DICOM file. It should be noted that DICOM files can come from x-rays, cone beam computed tomography (CBCT), magnetic resonance imaging (MRI), or any other in-depth medical study. However, CBCT images are the only files needed for the protocols described in this textbook, as all surgical planning programs demand this kind of DICOM file.

On the other side, implant surgery should be fully driven by the prosthetic plan. For that means, a digital image from patient dental arches is needed to set up said plan and later fabricate a template to reproduce it. Although CBCT images can give detailed information of tissue anatomy, surface definition of tooth and mucosa tends to be poor, especially at the occlusal level. Moreover, metal artifacts can cause great distortion over the images whenever present in the oral cavity. These are the main reasons why another file is needed, containing the external topography of the jaws. That is, a surface scan file, broadly known as STL file.

1.2 Surface Scans (STL Files)

Whenever there is a need of fabricating prosthetic restorations, surgical templates, or any other device that demands a correct fit in the oral cavity, jaw replicas are necessary to undertake said processes. Registration of the area of interest and its relation with neighboring teeth, opposing jaw and surrounding tissues is mandatory to develop a prosthetic plan to guide surgical protocols and then, fabricate a template to translate what has been digitally planned to the real-world scenario.

As stone casts have historically been used to work with, a necessity of a virtual model arises if wanting to do a digital planning. Therefore, a file that represents the surface geometry of a three-dimensional object has to be created [1]. Even though there is a huge variety of computer file extensions for 3D digital objects (such as .ply, .obj, .dcm), one specific file stands out among others, the .stl file (Fig. 1.1).

N. A. Rubio (✉)
Universidad de Buenos Aires,
Ciudad Autónoma de Buenos Aires, Argentina

© Springer Nature Switzerland AG 2021
J. M. Galante, N. A. Rubio (eds.), *Digital Dental Implantology*,
https://doi.org/10.1007/978-3-030-65947-9_1

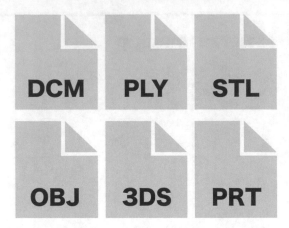

Fig. 1.1 Different file types for 3D objects

The original STL file was created for a vintage stereolithography CAD software by 3D Systems® Company in order to enhance data process for 3D printing and computer aided manufacturing. Despite originally been named as an abbreviation of "stereolithography", STL has also other backronyms, such as "Standard Tessellation Language" or "Standard Triangle Language", as it uses triangle forms to represent the shape of the object (Fig. 1.2). Nowadays, STL files are supported by many software programs and have become a universal CAD language. Contrary to this, some software systems utilize other file types to store data; some of them only valid within its own corresponding software (i.e., DCM file used by 3Shape®, Denmark; PLY used by Carestream®, USA), and some others may be used by multiple software packages (i.e., OBJ file). These files can store additional information, such as color, while this metadata is not present in an STL format (Fig. 1.2b).

Two methods for digitalizing patient dental arches are nowadays available: intraoral and extraoral scanning. On one hand, impression materials have been used to record teeth surfaces and its surrounding areas for a long period of time; improving accuracy, hydrophilic properties, and volume stability through time. Following this method, physical stone models can be created and then digitilized with an extraoral scanner to obtain a digital file. On the other hand, a direct digitalization of the oral cavity can be accomplished with intraoral scanners,

avoiding conventional impression techniques and thus, improving accuracy, saving time and easing patient experience (Fig. 1.3).

1.2.1 Intraoral Scanners

The implementation of intraoral scanners (IOS) in dentistry comes along with the development of CAD/CAM systems and enhances the digital workflow, providing fluency and precision. It also aims to reduce operative and treatment time, improve communication with laboratories, and reduce unnecessary storage space [2].

Optical, non-contact intraoral scanners are devices comparable to portable cameras used to record the surface of the oral topography. This camera needs to project a light (as it works in a dark environment) (Fig. 1.4) and record the oral situation within an integrated sensor, either as individual images or as a video. Different technologies are available for IOS, such as confocal imaging (iTero®, Netherlands), optical coherence tomography (E4D®, USA), or active wavefront sampling (3M True Definition®, USA) [3]. A description of all technologies used for scanner devices will not be addressed as it is not the purpose of this textbook. Although some scanners demand the use of powder-coating to reduce reflectivity, current tendency is to fabricate powder-free scanners to ease the scanning process and provide more comfort to the patient.

1.2.1.1 Scanning Technique. Tips and Recommendations

To assist data acquisition, some clinical tips may be stated:

– Use of retractor devices and moist control is recommended to get a better image. Some clinicians tend to switch the chair lamp off or dim the office light to avoid lighting interference [4]. Instruments used to separate oral tissues, such as mirrors, can be covered with a black nitrile finger glove (or similar) if metal reflection complicates the scanning process.
– Despite most systems have inbuilt heating elements to reduce fogging of the glass sur-

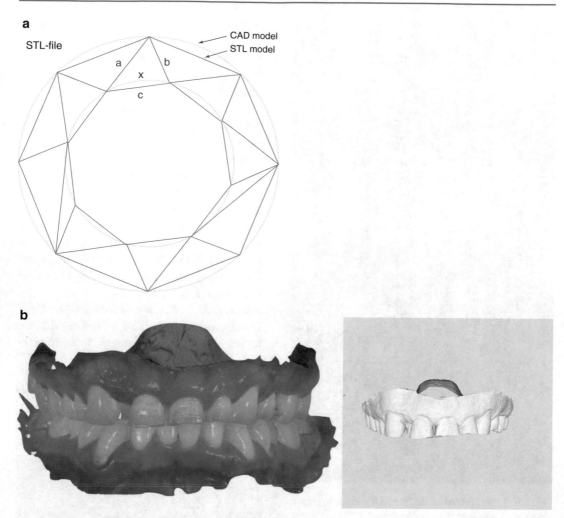

Fig. 1.2 (a) Standard Triangle Language (STL) stands for the reconstruction of an object based on triangular forms. (b) Surface scan in DCM format (left) and STL format (right). This DCM file is used by 3Shape® to add features such as color. When transforming this file into a plain STL file, only surface topography remains. Although not altered, the scan loses metadata

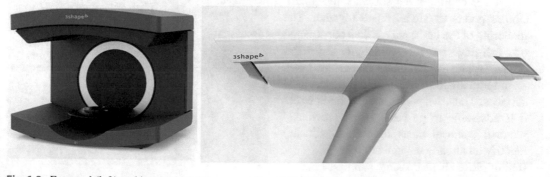

Fig. 1.3 Extraoral (left) and intraoral (right) scanners from 3 Shape®, Denmark

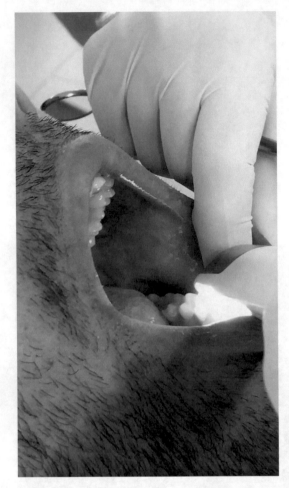

Fig. 1.4 Light emitted by the intraoral scanner to record the clinical situation

challenging; thus, conventional impression and extraoral scanning can be considered a suitable option in these cases.

- Some software may present a recommended scanning path to match its preset algorithms used to reconstruct the image. Deviation from the path may create inaccuracies in the data captured [5].
- Depending on the optical scanning technique employed, powder-coating with a titanium or magnesium dioxide powder may be required to enable the scanner capture the image. Latest IOS are designed powder-free to improve scanning experience. However, shiny metallic objects can disturb the process and so, may require some coating to capture the image (Fig. 1.5).
- Although it is not relevant for the overall outcome, continuous training with IOS will help reduce the number of images stored to com-

face that rests inside the scanner tip, moisture contamination or fogging can slow down the procedure.

- As data is captured, the software recognizes similar points to stitch images together. The rendering of the oral cavity is then constructed by merging images containing identical points. Typically, reference marks are taken from tooth anatomy, especially from occlusal surfaces. Thus, when the scanner loses track, it is advisable to go back to the previously scanned occlusal areas to let the software identify an already recognized spot.
- If multiple teeth are missing, soft tissue mobility can interfere with scanner recognition. Scanning Extended edentulous areas can be

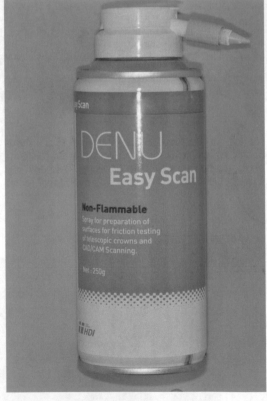

Fig. 1.5 Powder used to reduce reflectivity over shiny objects

plete the render. An efficient scanning technique will not only reduce operative time, but also reduce file processing time, improve computer performance, and minimize digital storage.

1.2.2 Extraoral Scanners

Dental technicians use a desktop laboratory scanner to digitalize stone casts or even conventional dental impressions. This turns out to be a perfect solution if not having an IOS in the dental office. Extraoral scanners (EOS) can be subdivided into two types: contact or contact-less. While the first refers to former digitalizing methods (i.e., Procera®, Nobel Biocare), non-contact or optical scanners are widely used today. Initially, contact or mechanical scanners used a probe to go across the object surface to detect its morphology. Naturally, the size of the probe and the angle of incidence influence scanning accuracy (Fig. 1.6).

Nowadays, optical scanners rely on a ray of light or laser to illuminate the object and collect information of the tridimensional surface using

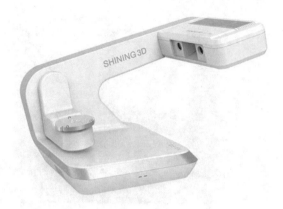

Fig. 1.7 Extraoral optical (non-contact) scanner. Autodesk® by Shining 3D

triangulation principles (Fig. 1.7). The light projected onto the object is reflected and captured by the receptor unit. The sensor measures the angle of the reflected light and so calculates the 3D data by means of triangulation principle (Fig. 1.8).

Since the model is exposed to a static light-emitting/light-receiving device, the rendering of the image is completed in a single plane. This offers the advantage of greater interpositional accuracy of the components within the model [5]. Thus, EOS are preferred in extended edentulous patients and full-arch reconstructions.

1.3 CBCT Images (DICOM Files)

DICOM comes from Digital Imaging and Communications in Medicine and it is considered to be the standard for sharing and management of medical imaging information and related data. In other words, DICOM is the extension file exported from a medical equipment after performing a study.

Most of the times, once image is acquired, the technician in charge of the study evaluates the outcome and assesses the visibility of relevant anatomic structures to dismiss the patient. Afterwards, the file containing the slices is processed by a software to determine jaw horizontal orientation, panoramic curve, and distribution of the axial slices. Said data processing, together with implant measurements, recognition of nerve canals and any other relevant information is

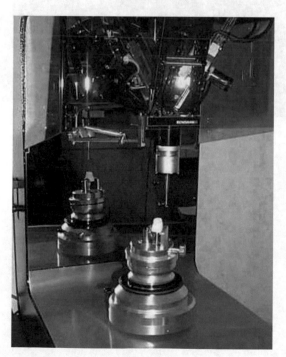

Fig. 1.6 Former contact scanners. Procera® by Nobel Biocare

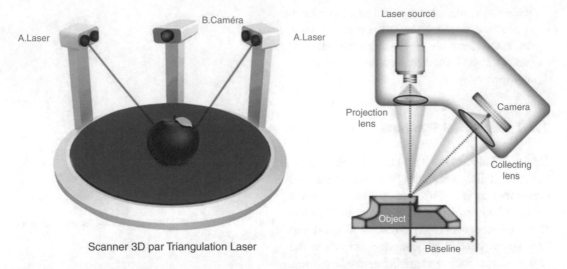

Scanner 3D par Triangulation Laser

Fig. 1.8 Triangulation principle. A light is projected over an object and the reflection is captured by a camera. The angle of reflection is measured to determine the surface of the scanned object

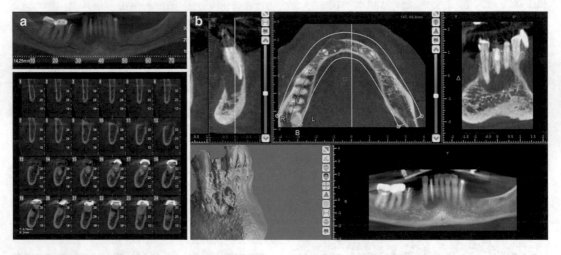

Fig. 1.9 CBCT visualization in conventional JPG file (**a**) and in software viewer (DICOM file manipulation). Panoramic curve, slices and 3D rendering can be custom-ized and the study can be navigated to get as much information as possible (**b**)

exported as a printable format (such as JPG or PNG files) and delivered to the patient (Fig. 1.9a).

Traditional implant planning usually relies on this processed image analysis to plan implant osteotomies. Nevertheless, additional surgical planning can be made by manipulating the file exported from the CBCT equipment. For that means, said file can be also delivered to the patient together with a CBCT basic software in a CD or USB portable device. The use of this viewer tends to be advantageous, as it offers more information than printed images and allows the professional to go across all slices and even simulate virtual implant placement (Fig. 1.9b).

Furthermore, the DICOM files contained in this CD/USB can be visualized either with the provided software or can be uploaded into a surgical planning software (Fig. 1.10). Each of these diagnostic options have its advantages and disadvantages, as it will be discussed in Chap. 2.

DICOM files can be often found in a folder named "images" or "data" inside the CD (Fig. 1.11). Also, these files can be sent by mail to avoid image printing and/or CD burning processes.

Fig. 1.10 Romexis® Viewer from Planmeca. This software comes together with CBCT images whenever a study is made with a Planmeca equipment. Additionaly, full version of this program can be purchased to unlock other features

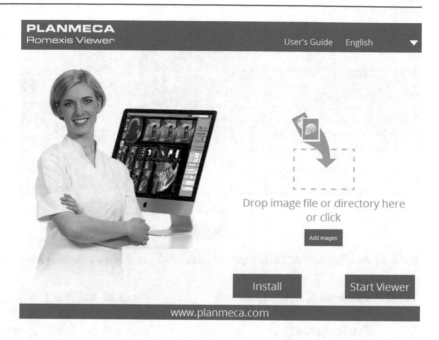

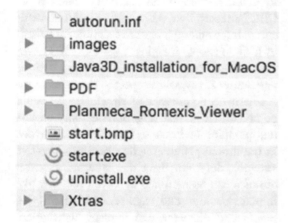

Fig. 1.11 Files contained in the CD that comes with the CBCT. The folder "images" gathers the slices that can be imported into any surgical planning software (DICOM files) while the icon "Start.exe" runs a viewer to visualize the study

DICOM files can be stored in three different formats (Fig. 1.12):

– DICOM (single frame): Every slice scanned by the CBCT equipment is saved in an independent file, resulting in multiple small size files. Software needs to put them all together to reconstruct the tridimensional image. Although apparently less pragmatic, this file exporting method is preferable over the other two as it pre-serves all relevant data and is supported by most software programs and viewers. However, this storage process increases study size and the parsing overhead as it replicates information in every file saved.

– DICOM (multi frame): This format was created to reduce file size and simplify parsing, storage, and communication, as it combines all slices into a single DICOM file. Nevertheless, some software do not support this format as they have not implemented it yet. Hopefully, this situation will revert to ease the digital workflow and global communication.

– DICOMDIR: It is a special file that serves as directory to a collection of DICOM files. This format is similar to a compressed ZIP/RAR file and can contain several studies from one or more patients, organized in the following way: Patient Level, Study Level, Series Level, Image Level. In hospitals or massive medical environments, DICOM Directory should theoretically shorten time required to find and display information stored when searching DICOM files. Still, this is not the case of our daily practice and not many imaging software support this file. A specific program can be downloaded from internet (often free of charge) to decompress info stored in the directory.

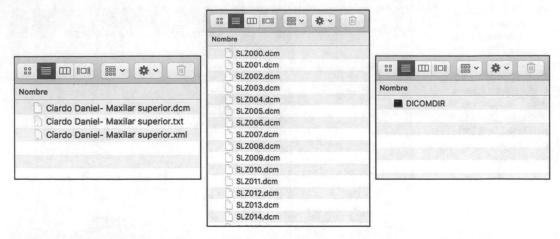

Fig. 1.12 Possible DICOM file storage: multi frame (left), single frame (center) and directory or DICOMDIR (right)

1.3.1 General Considerations for Justified Imaging Prescription

Any radiation exposure entails a risk to the patient. In concordance, it is essential that every radiographic examination shows a benefit to the patient [6]. The use of imaging modalities for pre-surgical dental implant planning should provide information supporting the following three goals: establish bone volume and quality, determine orientation of this bone in relation with the prosthetic plan, and identify anatomic or pathologic boundaries limiting implant placement [7]. Any study performed that does not deliver or add relevant information to the diagnosis should be avoided. This statement needs to be clear in order to understand that images must be carefully prescribed to prevent repeating the study and/or overexposing the patient.

According to the SEDENTEXCT Project [8], radiation doses, and hence risks, from dental Cone Beam Computed Tomography (CBCT) are generally higher than conventional dental radiography (intraoral or extraoral x-rays) but lower than Multi-Slice Computed Tomography (MSCT) scans. Overall, CBCT delivers better image quality and resolution compared with MSCT [9], which may also be important for fine detail of cortical bone thickness visualization [10]. Some studies suggest correlations between Hounsfield Units (HU) derived from CBCT scans and bone density, serving these images as predictors of implant stability [11]. Yet, other authors do not establish this measurement as trustworthy [12].

Awareness of relevant structures proximity could be one of the justifying premises for CBCT prescription. Although it would be difficult to trace among literature a significant benefit of tridimensional imaging, such as CBCT, over conventional two-dimensional imaging, such as panoramic X-ray, with respect to potential surgical harm to neurovascular structures, it should be noted that guided surgery relies only on virtual planning and data collected preoperatively. In traditional planning, whenever intraoperative situation does not meet the expectation, osteotomies can be modified to solve problems like implant position and angulation, implant type, length and diameter, and implant distribution. However, if a clinical situation does not meet a virtual planning, surgery is no longer driven by the virtual plan and has to be replaced by a free-hand protocol. Thus, it is mandatory to have trustworthy information of the underlying structures if wanting to set a guided approach. That is why a CBCT is always needed to perform the virtual surgery.

Optimization of radiation dose should follow the ALARA principle postulated by the International Commission on Radiology Protection (ICRP), which states that radiation dose should be kept as low as reasonably achievable (ALARA). Therefore, practitioners who prescribe or use CBCT units should ask for studies based on individual patient history and clinical examination and should specify exposure and image-quality parameters to achieve a proper diagnosis of the region of interest [13].

1.3.2 Techniques to Improve CBCT Imaging

Although prescribing a cone beam tomography tends to be a routine process, specifications on the demanded study can help the technician deliver a useful and high-quality tomography. As usual, good communication between professionals is mandatory. Thus, to optimize daily workflow, some details have to be taken into account.

1.3.2.1 Interarch Distance

Correct separation between the jaw of interest and its antagonist is of extreme importance.

Normally, a CBCT is performed while the patient is in occlusion and his/her chin rests on a mental support provided by the device. This allows the patient to remain still during the exam and avoid major deformation among images. This technique establishes an image in which upper and lower teeth are stitched together, with no space between them. Thus, occlusal surface and cusps cannot be distinguished properly (Figs. 1.13 and 1.14).

In order to compare and merge a surface scan of the jaw and a CBCT image from the same patient, tooth anatomy tends to be the best reference. For that means, separation between jaws allows the CBCT to give a neat image of the incisal edges and the occlusal surfaces. However, this image lacks of precision to make a virtual prosthodontic planning, a correct wax up, and a surgical template.

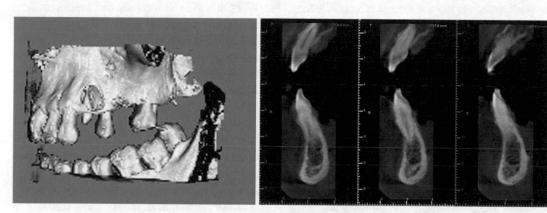

Fig. 1.13 Correct interarch separation allows visualization of the occlusal aspect of the teeth

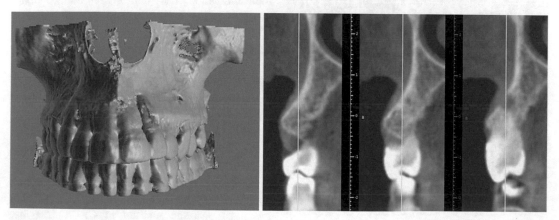

Fig. 1.14 Incorrect interarch separation. Occlusal surfaces are not visible

Sometimes, cotton rolls can serve as an occlusal stop to establish said interarch space. At least 10 mm distance is recommended and this can be hardly accomplished with only one roll. Other times, bite splints can be prepared previous to the CBCT. No specific jaw position needs to be addressed (i.e., centric relation registration) as correct occlusal relationship between arches will be present in surface scans. Bite registration materials can also interfere with tomography imaging. Though, it is important to evaluate possible material radiopaque properties.

Indications of interarch separation must be clearly stated on exam prescription.

1.3.2.2 Soft Tissue Separation

Indications on lips and cheeks displacement can help improve tooth, crestal bone and gingiva contour visualization. Usually, position of surrounding soft tissues is not considered when delivering a CBCT and lips and cheeks are in plain contact with jaw structures. Thus, delimitation between gingiva and neighboring oral mucosa is almost

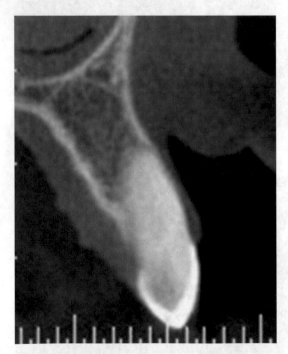

Fig. 1.15 Correct buccal tissue separation allows gingiva contour visualization. Usually, the tongue can be seen in plain contact with the palate. Instructions on tongue position can be useful to help assess the image merging process

impossible when inspecting the study. This is also present when the tongue rests over the palate and lingual aspect of the jaws (Fig. 1.15).

Correct diagnosis on crestal bone and gingiva thickness is useful when assessing an axial image in dental tomography. If the lip is displaced buccally, full contour of bone plates can be displayed to contribute with patient phenotype diagnosis, and considerations that comes ahead said diagnosis. Moreover, this contour visualization enhances the assessment of the image merging process, between surface scan and DICOM files (See 2.3 Image Merging Process).

Separation can be accomplished also with cotton rolls, but to ensure full tissue displacement, a lip retractor is preferred. Januário et al. [14] developed this novel method to improve buccal tissue visualization in order to measure its thickness and width using dental tomography and avoiding invasive techniques like bone sounding or transgingival probing (Fig. 1.16).

In summary, it is recommended to ask the technician to use a lip retractor and cotton rolls to perform the study. Instrument and materials can be provided to the patient when indicating a CBCT, just like when a radiographic template is delivered.

1.3.2.3 Field of View

The field of view (FoV) refers to the area of the patient that will be irradiated. In other words, it relates to the anatomic area that will be visualized on the study. Different FoV sizes can be used depending on the equipment and dental treatment indication. They can be divided into small, medium, or large:

- *Small FoV*: It covers around 6 in. diameter and allows proper visualization of 5 anterior or 3 posterior teeth. It is often used for endodontic purposes or to exam periodontal ligament, root fracture, periapical lesion, root canal morphology, and relation of an impacted tooth with the surrounding anatomical structures (Fig. 1.17).

It has the advantage of delivering high-quality image together with low 3D distortion, being the most accurate method in CBCT imaging. Equipments can either vary their fields of view to sat-

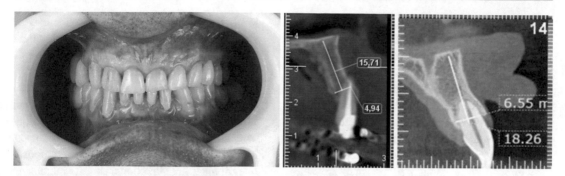

Fig. 1.16 Method published by Januário et al. [14] for soft tissue separation

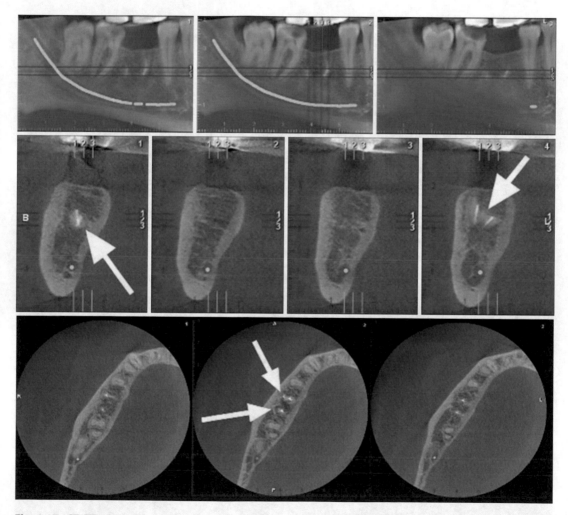

Fig. 1.17 CBCT taken with a small FoV. A small portion of the mandible can be assessed. Thus, image quality is improved and radiation dose is reduced

isfy every need or posses a fixed FoV. Thus, equipments having a fixed small FoV will require multiple scans to capture a complete arch, meaning more radiation to the patient. Therefore, multiple scans are superimposed to create a single image, which is usually seen as 3 circles superimposed in a horizontal view (one scan for the anterior region and one for each posterior zone) (Fig. 1.18).

– *Medium FoV*: It covers around 9 in. diameter; which is wide enough to visualize an entire arch with broad apical extension (Fig. 1.19). Usually, antagonist is seen up to bone crest

level. Dental elements of both arches can be seen if apical extension is reduced and patient is in occlusion. Nevertheless, visualization of one arch, correct apical extension, and inter-arch separation are recommended when indicating virtual planning protocols. Also, extension of this FoV allows display of adjacent cusps, to serve as merging references. Moreover, it can be used to diagnose temporo-mandibular joint alterations. Despite increasing the area of examination, whenever assessing implant placement, a medium FoV shows simi-

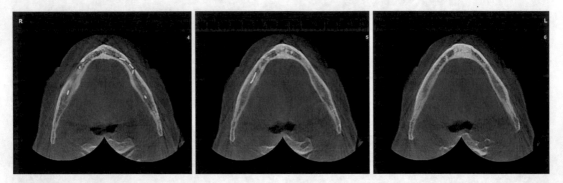

Fig. 1.18 A small FoV is used to get an image of the whole mandible. For that means, 3 separate scans are superimposed. Horizontal view shows three circles (scans) superimposed. Radiation dose is increased and so, a bigger FoV size is recommended in these cases

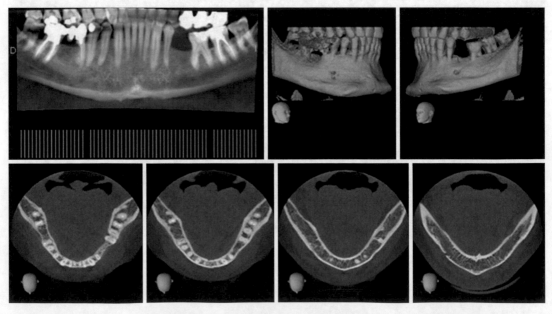

Fig. 1.19 Medium FoV can give an image of the whole jaw or maxilla. If arches are separated, opposing jaw is usually not visible

lar characteristics to a small one in terms of volume accuracy and image resolution [15].

- *Large FoV*: It covers around 12 in. diameter and is capable of delivering an image of the whole craniofacial area. This is especially useful in orthognathic surgery, skeletal anomalies, vast pathologies, or trauma cases. It can be also indicated to assess both jaws and contiguous regions, such as maxillary sinus, in one image (Fig. 1.20).

Implant planning can be accomplished successfully with every FoV size; however,

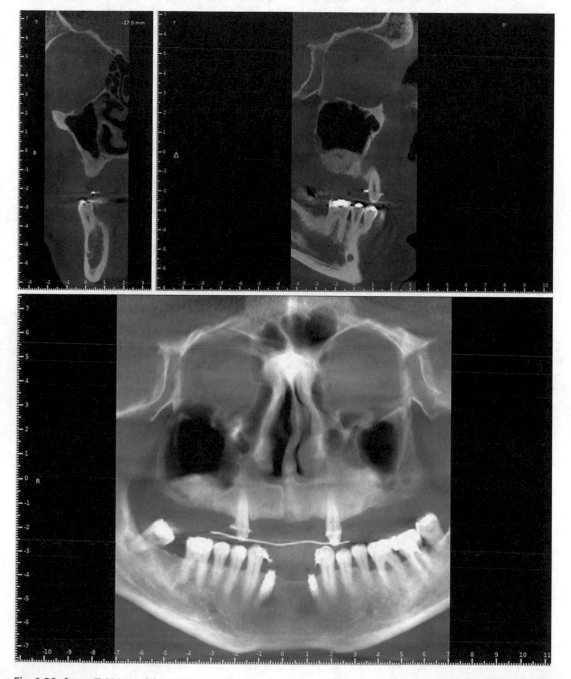

Fig. 1.20 Large FoV is useful to evaluate both arches and contiguous regions. Radiation with these scans is high, so cost-effect ratio should be analyzed carefully

major volume alterations can be expected when using a large FoV. Although said alterations should not affect conventional implant placement, virtual planning demands accuracy. Static guided surgery does not allow osteotomy modifications if bone topography does not resemble the CBCT image. Additionally, radiation dose should always be as low as possible. Therefore, large FoV indication should rely on cost-effect analyses (Fig. 1.21).

1.3.2.4 Voxel Size

A voxel is for the CBCT what the pixel is to an image. While a pixel is represented as a square (2 dimensions), a voxel is pictured as a cube (3 dimensions). The same concept known for a pixel works for a voxel: the smaller the pixel/voxel, the higher the quality of the image/CBCT. It can also be stated that, as the voxel become smaller, the detail captured in the study is higher, as well as time exposure and radiation dose. As a rule, smaller FoVs use smaller voxel sizes in order to obtain information from small structures. Thus, FoV indication comes along with voxel size unless otherwise specified. Such cases, as periodontal ligament changes, are not required for implant therapy analysis.

Additionaly, as smaller voxel sizes demand more exposure time, patients having difficulties remaining still might need faster scannings; meaning voxel size increment. As always, a balance between image quality and radiation dose has to be assessed.

1.3.3 Segmentation and 3D Reconstruction

Segmentation is the process used by a tomography software to separate one specific anatomic structure from the rest of the volume. This is a fundamental aspect of the CBCT, as virtual reconstructions help evaluate certain areas without other tissue interference. Segmentation comes along together with the process of 3D reconstruction, which involves the creation of a render from the gathering of sequential slices taken from the patient. This 3D reconstruction can be accomplished with or without selecting what tissue or area wants to be separated from the rest (segmentation). Surely, not selecting a specific tissue to be isolated will not deliver a neat image, as different tissues are superimposed.

Automatic segmentation is the most commonly used method and can be done in two ways: either by selecting a Hounsfield Unit (HU) threshold (each tissue has an average HU value) or by selecting a preset rendering configuration, previously defined by the software (Fig. 1.22).

Moreover, there are manual methods to accurately segment an area containing one or more tissues. These techniques vary among software programs but, in general aspects, clinician is guided through the slices to detect and select the area to be included in the reconstruction. Finally, a customized segmentation

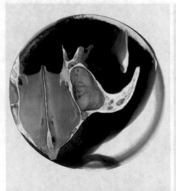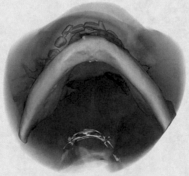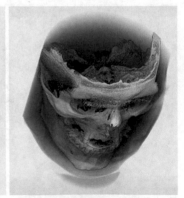

Fig. 1.21 Different FoV sizes. Small (left), medium (middle), and large (right). Radiation dose can be inferred from this representation

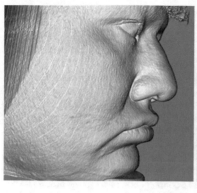
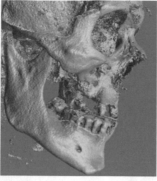
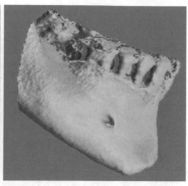

Fig. 1.22 Initial 3D reconstruction (left) with tissue superimposition (without segmentation); automatic segmentation by the HU delimitation process to visualize only hard tissue (middle), and customized segmentation to isolate a specific part of the mandible (right)

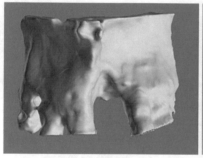
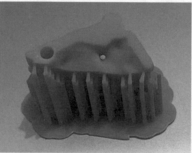
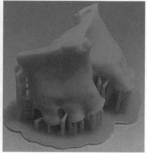

Fig. 1.23 Customized (advanced) segmentation and 3D printing of the surface model

is accomplished and a 3D rendering can be visualized.

As a final step, the render can be exported as a surface image (STL file) either to be manipulated in other software or to be printed by an additive method (3D printing) to obtain a stereolithographic model (Fig. 1.23). This process will be discussed in Part II.

References

1. Alghazzawi TF. Advancements in CAD/CAM technology: options for practical implementation. J Prosthodont Res. 2016;60(2):72–84.
2. Richert R, Goujat A, Venet L, Viguie G, Viennot S, Robinson P, Farges JC, Fages M, Ducret M. Intraoral scanner technologies: a review to make a successful impression. J Healthc Eng. 2017;2017:8427595.
3. Al-Hassimy H, Al-Hassimy H, Al-Hassimy A. Review of the intraoral scanners at IDS 2019. Cologne: Institute of Digital Dentistry.
4. Revilla-León M, Jiang P, Sadeghpour M, Piedra-Cascón W, Zandinejad A, Özcan M, Krishnamurthy VR. Intraoral digital scans: Part 2-influence of ambient scanning light conditions on the mesh quality of different intraoral scanners. J Prosthet Dent. 2020;124(5):575–80. pii: S0022–3913(18)30995–8.
5. Galucci G, Evans C, Tahmseb A. ITI treatment guide, vol. 11. Berlin: Quintessence Publishing; 2019.
6. Harris D, Horner K, Gröndahl K, Jacobs R, Helmrot E, Benic GI, Bornstein MM, Dawood A, Quirynen M. E.A.O. guidelines for the use of diagnostic imaging in implant dentistry 2011. A consensus workshop organized by the European Association for Osseointegration at the Medical University of Warsaw. Clin Oral Implants Res. 2012;23(11):1243–53.
7. Bornstein M, Scarfe W, Vaugh V, Jacobs R. Cone beam computed tomography in implant dentistry: a systematic review focusing on guidelines, indications and radiation dose risks. Int J Oral Maxillofac Implants. 2014;29(suppl):55–77.
8. Horner K, Armitt G et al. Cone Beam CT for dental and maxillofacial radiology. Evidence-Based Guidelines. Radiation Protection No. 172. European Commission ISSN 1681–6803.

9. Loubele M, Guerrero ME, Jacobs R, Suetens P, van Steenberghe D. Comparison of jaw dimensional and quality assessments of bone characteristics with cone-beam CT, spiral tomography, and multi-slice spiral CT. Int J Oral Maxillofac Implants. 2007;22:446–54.

10. Razavi T, Palmer RM, Davies J, Wilson R, Palmer PJ. Accuracy of measuring the cortical bone thickness adjacent to dental implants using cone beam computed tomography. Clin Oral Implants Res. 2010;21:718–25.

11. Aranyarachkul P, Caruso J, Gantes B, Schulz E, Riggs M, Dus I, Yamada JM, Crigger M. Bone density assessments of dental implant sites: 2. Quantitative cone-beam computerized tomography. Int J Oral Maxillofac Implants. 2005;20:416–24.

12. Bryant JA, Drage NA, Richmond S. Study of the scan uniformity from an i-CAT cone beam computed tomography dental imaging system. Dentomaxillofac Radiol. 2008;37:365–74.

13. Pauwels R, Araki K, Siewerdsen JH, Thongvigitmanee SS. Technical aspects of dental CBCT: state of the art. Dentomaxillofac Radiol. 2015;44(1):20140224.

14. Januário AL, Barriviera M, Duarte WR. Soft tissue cone-beam computed tomography: a novel method for the measurement of gingival tissue and the dimensions of the dentogingival unit. J Esthet Restor Dent. 2008;20(6):366–73.

15. Hedesiu M, Baciut M, Baciut G, Nackaerts O, Jacobs R, SEDENTEXCT Consortium. Comparison of cone beam CT device and field of view for the detection of simulated periapical bone lesions. Dentomaxillofac Radiol. 2012;41(7):548–52.

CAD: Computer-Assisted Design

2

Nicolás A. Rubio

2.1 Introduction

In digital implant dentistry, two different kinds of software packages can be found. Therefore, each dental program can be catalogued either as a prosthetic planning software or an implant planning software. While the first ones are used mainly by dental labs, the second ones are used by clinicians to visualize CBCT images, plan implant placement, and design surgical templates.

An implant planning software allows the surgeon to navigate the tomography through the slices and personalize its visualization. Panoramic curve, distance between slices, bone density threshold, brightness and contrast are examples of parameters that can be customized by these programs. Moreover, virtual implants can be placed to make the most out of the surgical plan.

Finally, after diagnosis and virtual implant placement is achieved, a surgical template can be fabricated to reproduce said planning during surgery. This template can be designed by making use of a virtual cast taken from the patient, in order to be supported by teeth, mucosa, or even bone structures.

Implant brand, model, length and diameter can be selected from software library. Drilling system usually comes along with implant selection, but sometimes can be modified. Thus,

N. A. Rubio (✉)
Universidad de Buenos Aires,
Ciudad Autónoma de Buenos Aires, Argentina

instruments used to perform the desired surgery will depend on software settings.

Understanding the design itself helps clinician recognize the importance of the data collection process that takes place previously. Fortunately, learning curve tends to be more easygoing with implant planning software rather than with prosthetic planning software, as surgeons are normally familiarized with tomography viewers.

2.2 Planning Software

Even though both programs (prosthetic and surgical software) are basically CAD programs (as they are set to design), the term "CAD software" in dentistry normally refers to the group of technology used to design restorations, bite splints, abutments, and other prosthetic elements. It is important to differentiate between prosthetic planning software (Fig. 2.1) and implant planning software (Fig. 2.2). In this textbook, focus will be made on programs that allows the visualization of CBCT images and the design of a virtual surgical procedure, that is, implant planning software.

As described in Chap. 1, two types of files are managed in these programs, one to assess bone anatomy (DICOM file taken from CBCT images) (Fig. 2.3) and one to perform the prosthetic design and fabricate a template for guided surgery (STL file or equivalent taken from intraoral or extraoral surface scanners) (Fig. 2.4). Thus, if

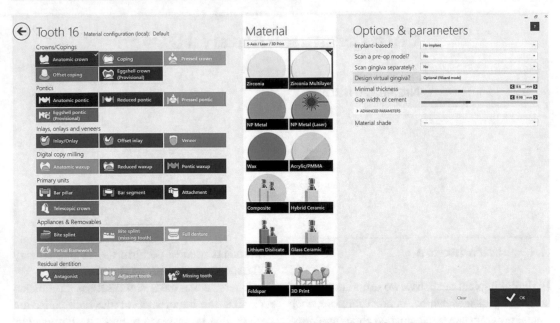

Fig. 2.1 Job definition in a prosthetic planning software (CAD program, Exocad®, GmbH)

Fig. 2.2 Job definition in an implant planning software (CBCT viewer and virtual implant placement program, Implant Studio®, 3Shape)

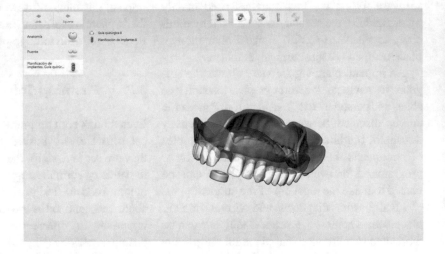

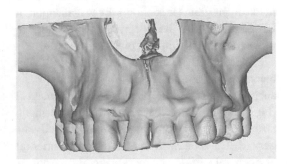

Fig. 2.3 DICOM file from patient CBCT

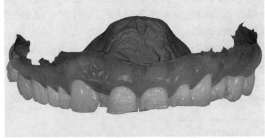

Fig. 2.4 Surface scan from patient oral situation. This DCM file contains additional information, such as color, and can be transformed into a conventional STL file

only a DICOM file is uploaded in an implant planning software, clinician will be able to navigate the study, measure distances or place a virtual implant, but won't be able to determine a precise prosthetic plan (digital wax-up and future crown position) or even deliver a surgical template [1].

As simple as it sounds, each file allows a job to be made and so, both are needed to get the most out of the software. Complete patient diagnosis involves getting all the information from patient initial situation to anticipate intraoperative risks, evaluate site conditions, and determine the best treatment option for the patient. Getting involved into the digital world implies gathering more patient information, spending more time on the preoperative phase to improve diagnosis in order to reduce clinical time and deliver more predictable treatments.

2.2.1   Available Software

In the market we can easily come across with different software options: free demo programs, which are usually called "viewers", open-source software and full version programs.

- *Tomography Viewers*: usually, they come with data delivered to the patient in a CD/portable device, together with the study. Depending on the tomography equipment used, a free version of the same brand is provided; i.e., Planmeca® equipments use Romexis® Viewer, a compact version of a broader planning software that only allows navigation through the tomography (Fig. 2.5). Additionally, full version of Romexis® software can be purchased to access all features. Moreover, the same files that are visualized in the corresponding viewer can be imported to a third-party software, thanks to the described universal language: the DICOM file.

- *Open-source software*: broadly used nowadays, free implant planning software can be downloaded from internet and offer a huge variety of tools. They are a very good option to enter the digital world as they require almost no cost and allow the clinician to navigate DICOM files, perform a simple wax-up to serve as prosthetic plan, place virtual implants, and attach surface scans to design a surgical template. In summary, surgeons can get more information with these programs than with traditional asseesment of printed

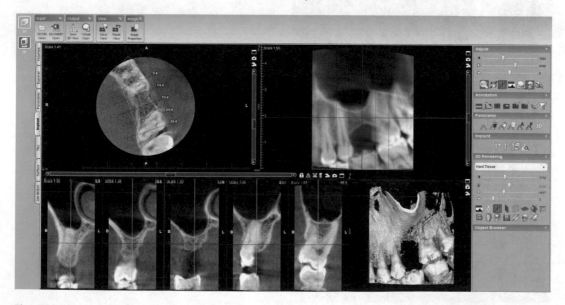

Fig. 2.5 Romexis® CBCT viewer from Planmeca

images or conventional tomography viewers, without falling into any costs. The software permits template fabrication to go into a fully guided surgical procedure but charge to export said design. To clarify, in order to obtain an STL file to manufacture the template with a CAM procedure, the program needs to export the file. Although planning is free of charge, exporting files is not. This action would be comparable to designing a presentation on PowerPoint or Keynote, so to practice the lecture, without being able to save the project and actually reproducing it with a projector.

Nevertheless, the cost of exporting files is low and can be a good option to get inside the digital planning environment without almost any investment. Perhaps the most known and used free program is BlueSkyBio® (Fig. 2.6).

- *(Full Version Programs - Purchased) Implant Planning Software*: The above described open-source software has limitations, such as poor tooth wax-up, and advantages, such as multiple surface scans uploading, CBCT customized segmentation and combination of different drilling systems. However, unexperienced dentists can easily get lost among the

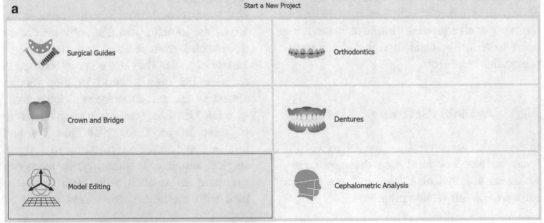

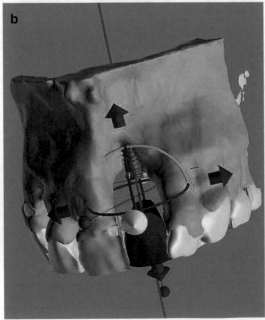

Fig. 2.6 Virtual implant planning with an open source software (BlueSkyPlan 4® from BlueSkyBio) (**a, b**)

many features and combinations offered by these programs. Moreover, multiple designing options can incur into errors and potential risks for the surgical guided treatment [2]. Therefore, advance interfaces are offered in full version programs, where an easygoing protocol leads the clinician into a path that begins with file uploading and finalizes with template design. Normal values are preset to assure good clinical performance and warning signs alert the user from potential misfits or surgical risks (Fig. 2.7). Graphics are enhanced and the planning experience is more friendly (Fig. 2.8). At the end of the path, an STL file is delivered for the guide to be manufactured (Fig. 2.9). Although the overall

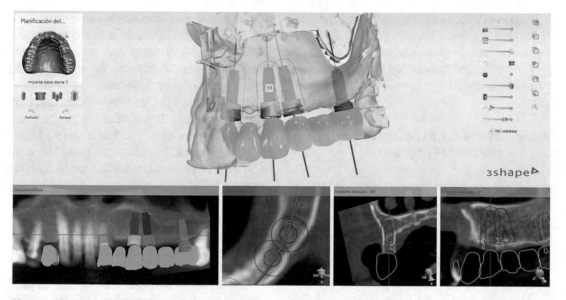

Fig. 2.7 Implant proximity alert is clearly visualized (red) while proper distance is approved (green). Default distance parameters can be customized for each clinical case

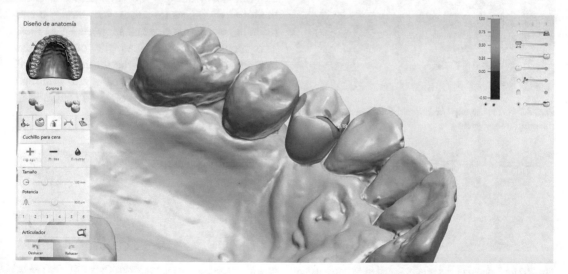

Fig. 2.8 Virtual wax-up, adjacent tooth and antagonist proximity, cusp heights and occlusal surface can be easily assessed

designing process is usually straightforward, few customizations can be accomplished in some of these software. In summary, they offer high quality image and a friendly interface to minimize potential errors and deliver a controlled outcome, but some of them do not permit modifications to the implant planning protocol; i.e., an implant osteotomy cannot be performed with a customized or different drilling system; nor can the tomography be segmented to create bone stereolithographic models. In this category, you can find programs like: Implant Studio® from 3Shape®; CoDiagnostix® from Dental Wings®; Exoplan® from GmBh®.

2.2.2 Interactions Between Software Programs

As described previously, communication between software depends exclusively on the usage of the same language. It is important to understand that, even though there is a universal language sup-

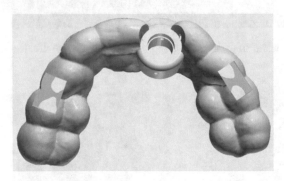

Fig. 2.9 STL file exported from the software to fabricate the surgical template

ported by all software (standard tessellation language or STL), each program can use its own language; i.e., 3Shape software uses DCM files. This provokes that both files are supported and so, can be uploaded to plan the surgery (Fig. 2.10). However, after implant planning is completed, the software delivers an STL file containing the template to be manufactured, but preserves all planning information (surface scan with the virtual wax-up and implant position) in its own specific language. Although this semi-open system allows communication between programs, some information is lost in each communication. The same inconvenience can be seen between implant and prosthetic software.

To give an example, if using a 3Shape Implant Studio® software, the surface scan can be uploaded either with a STL file or with a DCM file (taken from a Trios Scanner from 3Shape). DCM will carry additional information such as color and STL file will lose all additional information other than the surface topography (Fig. 2.11). After finalizing the design, a template will be exported in a universal language (STL). Moreover, the file that represents the modified surface scan (jaw and implant) will be exported in DCM format. This means that, in order to proceed with a full digital prosthetic treatment, like fabricating a provisional crown for immediate implant loading, you will need a prosthetic CAD software from the same brand (3Shape) or anyone else that supports DCM files. The modified surface scan file contains the implant in its position and the virtual wax-up of the prosthetic plan, both necessary to continue with the digital workflow to obtain a restoration.

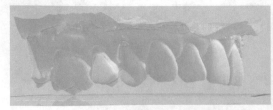
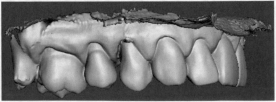

Fig. 2.10 Same object digitally stored in different extension files. PLY file (left) obtained with Emerald® scanner from Planmeca and STL file (right) compatibility. Both files are exported from the scanner. Only STL file can be uploaded in a 3Shape software as it only supports STL (universal language) and DCM (its own language)

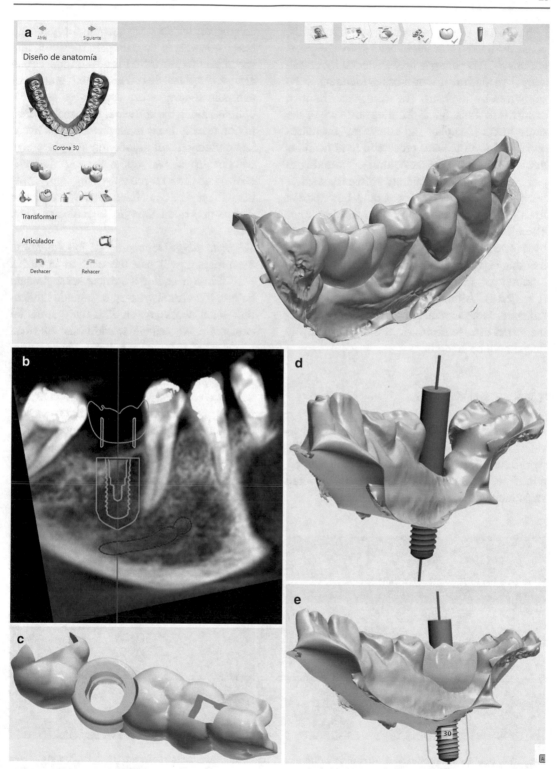

Fig. 2.11 Same clinical case as Fig. 2.10 is uploaded using a compatible format (STL). Virtual wax-up (**a**) and implant planning (**b**) are performed. Template is exported into an STL file to be printed or milled (**c**) and information of implant position (**d**) and crown wax-up used to fabri-cate a restoration (**e**) are only exported in DCM files. Thus, complete brand software package (both surgical and prosthetic programs) is needed to generate a dynamic workflow

The same example can be given backwards, when using for instance, Exocad software (most common CAD software used in dental labs nowadays) to design a crown/bridge/denture to be supported by implants. The design can be then exported to the surgical planning software of the same brand (Exoplan®) to allow implant placement and simultaneous prosthetic modifications in a synergic way. On the contrary, if wanting to use another surgical planning software, such as DDS Pro®, a new STL file should be exported from Exocad, containing the restorations. Therefore, initial surface scan would be replaced by this new model. Clinician should keep in mind that this new model has to provide enough information to merge with the CBCT image (Fig. 2.12). Although possible, this technique demands more experience on software management and creates obstacles in a digital pathway that should be smooth.

2.2.3 CAD Workflow

Although every CAD program has its own characteristics, all systems offer the user a similar workflow [3]. Once understood the path needed, clinicians can easily use any software. Overall steps include:

– *Job definition*: This can seem an insignificant task but has all to do with path selection. Site specifications regarding crown/bridge virtual design, implant distribution and guided or non-guided surgery are usually the available options among the software. Incorrect job definition usually leads to an unwanted pathway, i.e.: defining a non-guided implant placement without virtual wax-up, will make the software avoid the STL file uploading step; as this file will only be demanded whenever template design or virutal wax-up is indicated (Fig. 2.13).
– *File uploading*: Depending on job definition, the program will ask the user to upload a CBCT image and/or a surface scan. As said before, if a virtual wax-up or a guide fabrication is not necessary, an STL file will not be demanded. Nevertheless, additional files can be uploaded to have more patient information (Fig. 2.14).
– *File cropping*: This step reduces volume information, especially in extended DICOM images, helping the clinician focus on site evaluation and also reducing memory used to navigate and store the project. Special attention should be kept on leaving enough dental structures in the cropped DICOM file to merge with the STL (Fig. 2.15).

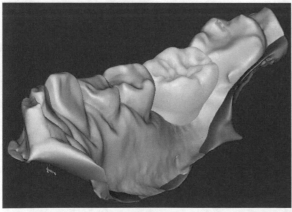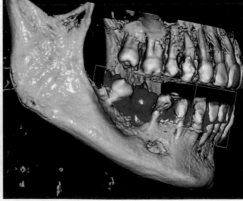

Fig. 2.12 Same clinical case is used to explain a different software interaction. First, the surface scan is uploaded in a CAD software (Exocad®) and a crown is waxed up (left). Second, a new file is exported (model and crown design) in STL format. Finally, this latest file is imported into a surgical planning software (DDS Pro®) and adjacent teeth are used to merge the CBCT and the new surface scan (right). Note that the waxed-up tooth is not present in the DICOM file. Multiple reference points are present in this case, so software interaction is possible

Fig. 2.13 Job definition. In this case, tooth #14 indication is stablished. Wax-up function is selected (will require upper jaw surface scan and antagonist) for single implant virtual placement (will require patient CBCT) and template fabrication for static guided surgery (will require upper jaw surface scan)

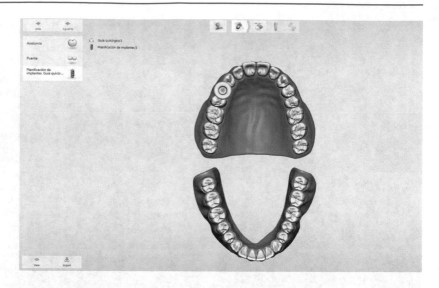

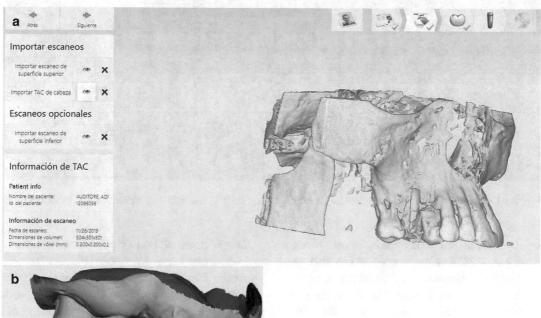

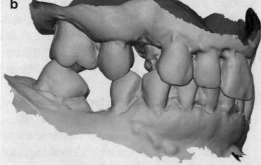

Fig. 2.14 CBCT (**a**) and both jaw scans (**b**) are uploaded according to job definition

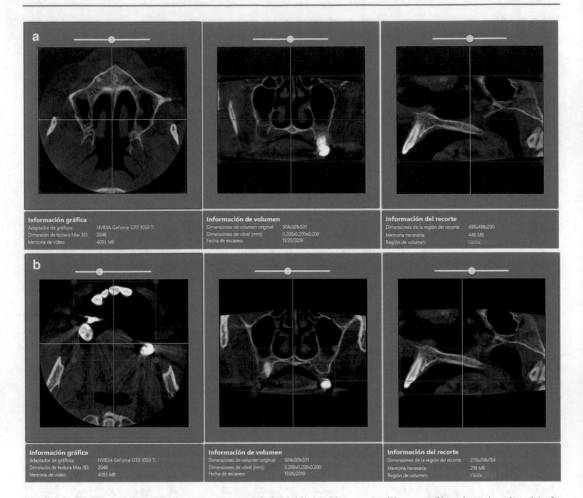

Fig. 2.15 CBCT cropping. Computer memory needed (highlighted in green) will vary as file volume is reduced (**a**, **b**)

– *Panoramic curve definition*: when examining a CBCT, a panoramic curve that goes throw the center of the bone ridge at a crestal level has to be drawn. This serves for determining the axial views where the virtual implant will be placed (Fig. 2.16).

– *Mental nerve definition*: Whenever planning an implant in the mandible, this is a necessary step to verify implant security distance during its placement.

– *Virtual Wax-Up*: Positioning a tooth provided by the library and adapting it to the desired clinical situation comes prior to implant placement, as the intention of this protocol is to deliver an implant that is prosthetically driven. This step can appear before or after CBCT

image manipulation (crop, panoramic curve and mental nerve definition) (Fig. 2.17).

– *Image Merging*: While some programs offer automatic matching, this step usually requires identifying anatomical points present in both STL and DICOM files. Correct merging is one of the key steps for achieving a good outcome (Fig. 2.18).

– *Implant Placement*: Implant selection and positioning throughout CBCT axial slices, together with emergence profile assessment towards the future crown demands same expertise as conventional implant placement. Main advantage here is the possibility to change implant brand/model or length/diameter to fit into the clinical situation. Also, a

Fig. 2.16 Panoramic curve definition to visualize axial slices

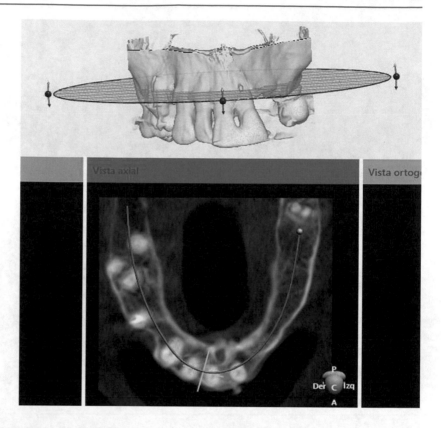

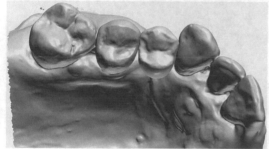

Fig. 2.17 Tooth wax-up

tomized, such as space between guide and teeth (fit), distance from implant platform to sleeve (offset), material (guide) thickness, manufacturing configurations (DLP, SLA, milling system) and space between guide and sleeve. Also, other items can be added to the template, such as exploring windows to assess correct fitting, bars or reinforcement structures and other written references (i.e.: name of the patient or other relevant information). Every aspect of the template design has to be analyzed in relation to the manufacturing method and material.

safety perimeter is preset within the software to detect possible proximity to nerves or adjacent implants. These values can be modified to customize the surgical approach (Fig. 2.19).

– *Guide Fabrication*: As with conventional splints, retentive areas should be avoided in order to properly fit the template. So, insertion axis is determined within the software to visualize these areas and draw the contour of the future guide (Fig. 2.20). In this step, some values can be cus-

– *Confirmation and File Export*: Normally, a surgical report containing the drilling sequence and the virtual planning is delivered to the user (or the surgeon if designed by a third party), to be checked and confirmed (Fig. 2.21). Afterwards, an STL file is exported containing the information necessary for milling or printing the template. For legal motives, some programs do not allow the user to modify the surgical plan after project is confirmed. Additionally, a list of materials needed for the

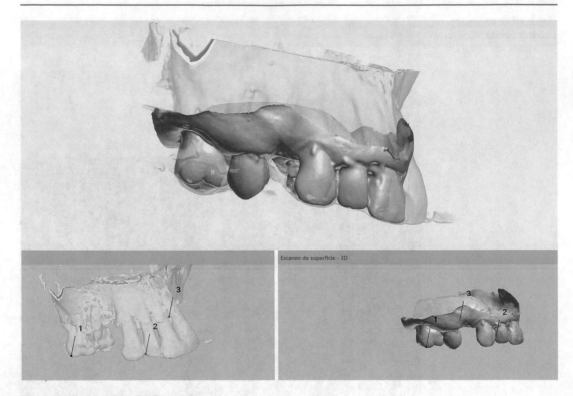

Fig. 2.18 Fusion of the CBCT and the surface scan

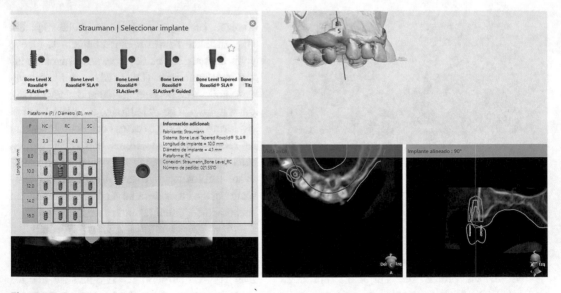

Fig. 2.19 Implant selection and security margin assessment can be done in multiple views to ensure a correct outcome

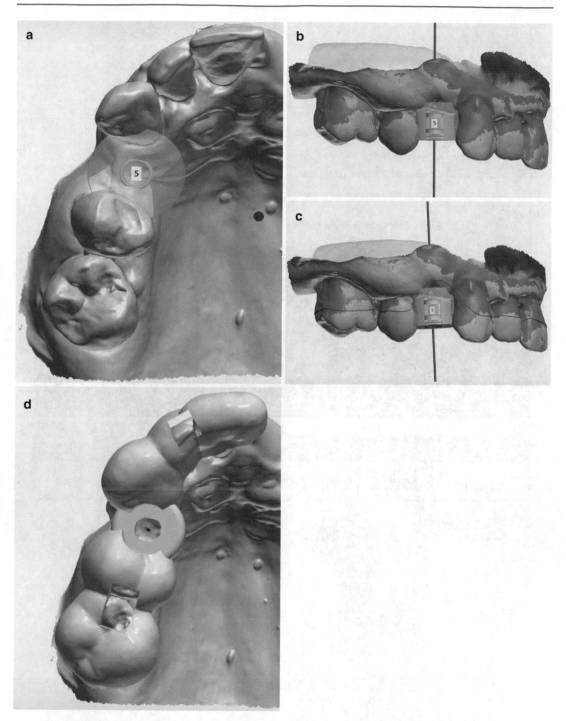

Fig. 2.20 Guide fabrication. Insertion axis determination from an occlusal view (**a**). Shadow areas indicate retentive zones to be avoided with the design (**b**). Guide contour delimitation (**c**) and inspection windows added to assess proper fit (**d**)

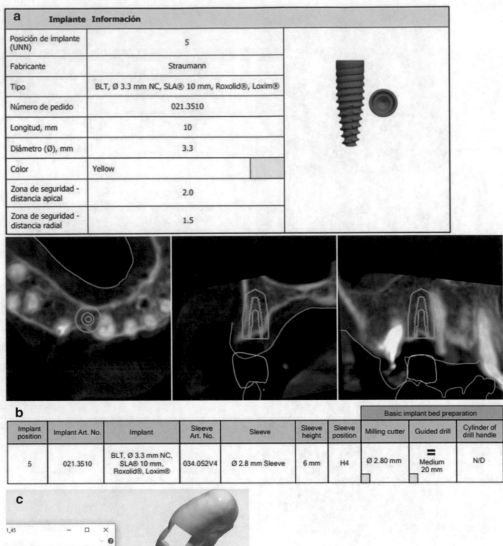

a	Implante Información	
Posición de implante (UNN)	5	
Fabricante	Straumann	
Tipo	BLT, Ø 3.3 mm NC, SLA® 10 mm, Roxolid®, Loxim®	
Número de pedido	021.3510	
Longitud, mm	10	
Diámetro (Ø), mm	3.3	
Color	Yellow	
Zona de seguridad - distancia apical	2.0	
Zona de seguridad - distancia radial	1.5	

b							Basic implant bed preparation		
Implant position	Implant Art. No.	Implant	Sleeve Art. No.	Sleeve	Sleeve height	Sleeve position	Milling cutter	Guided drill	Cylinder of drill handle
5	021.3510	BLT, Ø 3.3 mm NC, SLA® 10 mm, Roxolid®, Loxim®	034.052V4	Ø 2.8 mm Sleeve	6 mm	H4	Ø 2.80 mm	Medium 20 mm	N/D

c

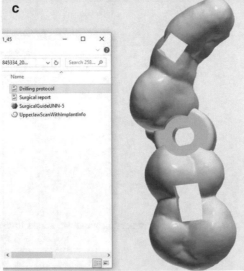

Fig. 2.21 Surgical and drilling reports (**a**, **b**). Surgical guide finalized and file exportation (**c**). Note that surgical and drilling reports are exported in PDF files to be visualized or printed. Additionally, surgical template is exported in a universal STL format to be milled or printed (see Chap. 3) while information about implant position is exported in a specific file type (DCM file), used only by 3Shape software (see Sect. 2.2.2)

surgery itself is detailed. This includes: implants, drills and sleeves needed to perform the surgery as planned.

2.3 Image Merging Process

Perhaps the most decisive and meticulous step in the whole digital implant planning pathway is the fusion between CBCT image (DICOM file) and surface scan (STL file or similar). As said before, the planning is performed in a dual way: placing the virtual implant in the bone by visualizing the CBCT and transposing its position to the patient by designing a template which guides the osteotomy. The template has to be designed from a neat model; thus, teeth and mucosa reconstruction from a CBCT image cannot be used as a virtual cast, as it lacks of accuracy. For that means, a surface scan is needed.

Therefore, if virtual implant placement is planned on one image (DICOM file) and guide is designed on another image (STL file), these two images have to be carefully related.

It is important to highlight that errors committed during the image merging process will not stop the digital workflow; as this will continue and the error will be transferred to the surgery. Implant will be placed on the CBCT image and the guide successfully designed. The template will certainly fit but the position of the drills will not represent the designed osteotomy. This is an important fact to rationalize, because the clinician will not be aware of this error until osteotomy is already made.

Image merging usually involves two steps, marking points in both images to direct the merging recognition and manual adjustment. Depending on the clinical situation, the points detected can be either anatomic teeth structures or radiopaque indicators.

2.3.1 3-Point Recognition (Automatic Alignment)

Whenever dental structures are conserved, anatomic crowns are used to stablish alignment points. For that means, a double window pops up, showing the user the surface model and the tridimensional reconstruction of the CBCT (3D rendering). Three points, situated as far of each other as possible, are selected in both windows (Fig. 2.22). Alignment can be automatically proposed by the software if images are both neat and contain enough preserved tooth structures. This is the case of the most sophisticated software programs. Nevertheless, manual point determination can help the software compare and match tooth shapes. Although an easy task, some considerations can be taken into account to improve the matching process:

– *Tissue Density*: it is important to adjust density threshold to correctly visualize enamel, bone, and cementum while erasing soft tissue. Hounsfield Unit (HU) is the value that needs

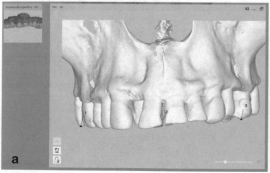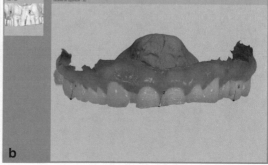

Fig. 2.22 Selection of 3 points in each image to start the automatic merging process (**a, b**)

to be adjusted in order to select tissue density. Soft tissue separation, indicated in CBCT prescription, helps distinguish different tissues with accuracy (Fig. 2.23).

- *Magnification and Orientation*: Stablishing precise dots is the goal; so, magnifying the image can help determine a precise location of the selected spot to be compared and merged. Moreover, clinician should try to be equally accurate in both images. Thus, image size and orientation should be adjusted as similar as possible during every spot selection (Fig. 2.24).
- *Cusps selection*: cervical aspects of the teeth, such as zenith points, are not the best matching material, as they can be determined clearly only in the surface model. HU value is normally set to hide soft tissue and so, gingival

margin is not visualized. Additionally, proximal areas are not neat spots to rely on within CBCT reconstruction as image from adjacent enamels can be superimposed. Buccal cusps, especially tips, are the main choice for this procedure (Fig. 2.25). Natural teeth are preferred to jacket crowns. Metal objects are not matching material due to the image scattering that results from tomography artifacts.

2.3.2 Manual Adjustment

Following the comparison of the stablished points and the merging of the images, an inspection of the result has to take place. On some software, a colored scale of matching values uses a Boolean difference process to show the result of the

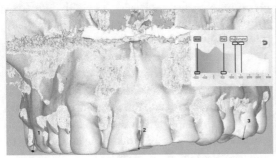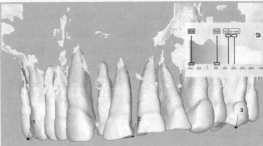

Fig. 2.23 A low-density threshold configuration (left) will generate a scattered image and soft tissue interference will hinder the fusion of the two images. A high-density threshold setup (right) will certainly erase bone topogra-

phy and leave tooth structure, especially in the maxilla. Nevertheless, superficial tooth anatomy can be potentially blurred if threshold is adjusted too high

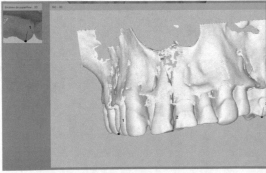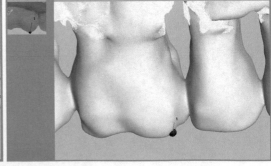

Fig. 2.24 Different angulation and magnification can confuse the clinician. A dot is selected to resemble the dot position in the surface scan (tooth number 16) using a dif-

ferent view (left). When amplifying and rotating the image, the clinician can appreciate the dot misposition (right)

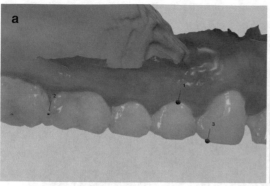

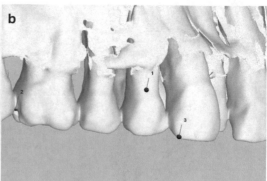

Fig. 2.25 Proximal areas are zones of conflict because of image superimposition within the CBCT (dot 2); cervical areas are also not distinguishable in the CBCT as soft tis-sue is erased in this step (dot 1). Cusps are the areas of election (dot 3) (**a**, **b**)

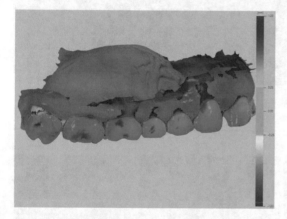

Fig. 2.26 Matching of around 0.25 mm is corroborated with a colored scale

merging process (Fig. 2.26). This tool helps identify zones of mismatch in order to correct them.

Even if not having this tool available, the confirmation protocol involves scrolling through the CBCT slices to observe the surface scan contour in relation to the tomography. STL file is shown as a hint image to improve this assessment (Fig. 2.27).

If merging process is not successfully achieved, new alignment points can be used (sometimes more points can be added) to correct positioning. Furthermore, the surface scan can be manipulated, moved and rotated to fit the desired position. This is useful in cases where few tooth structures and extended edentulous areas represent zones of mismatch. In said cases, options like extra radiopaque indicators can be a good solution. However, in absence of these indicators, palate and adjacent attached and firm mucosa are used to verify and manually adjust the position of the scan. Again, soft tissue separation during the CBCT study gives the clinician a good gingiva contour visualization.

Manual adjustment has to be left as an ultimate solution, whenever failing to merge images properly by using alignment points or not being able to count on extra indicators.

2.3.3   Extra Radiopaque Indicators

Extended edentulous spaces, such as one posterior quadrant absence, can be detrimental to the merging process. In these cases, a tomographic template can be used to deliver one or more radiopaque spots to serve as alignment points. As these points have to be also present in the surface model, the scanning process has to collect information of the patient jaw using the device. It is recommended to perform a notch in the template and do the scan before filling it with radiopaque material. This way the notch visualized in the surface scan will correspond to the radiopaque dot visualized on the tomography (Fig. 2.28).

It is important to remember that both STL and DICOM files have to contain the same information; that is, if the patient is going to use a tomographic template, the intraoral/extraoral scan should be performed using that template.

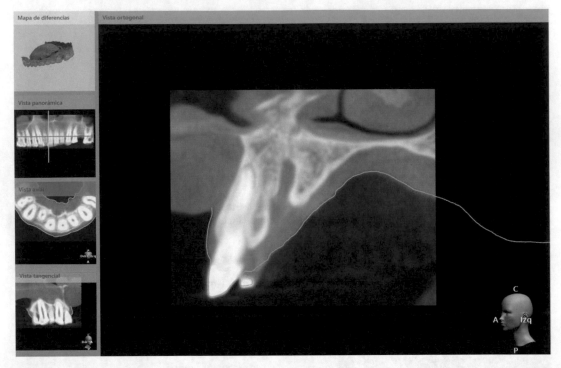

Fig. 2.27 A hint of the surface scan is superimposed to the CBCT slices. Soft tissue separation helps the assessment, as the contour of the gingival and palate can be easily distinguished

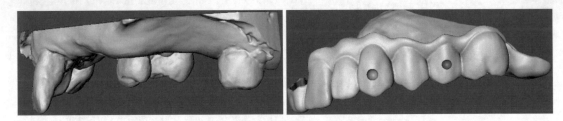

Fig. 2.28 Patient initial situation (left) and radiographic template digitally designed (right). Notches in teeth #23 and #25 are fabricated to be filled with radiopaque material and serve as extra alignment points

2.3.4 Image Merging Process in Edentulous Patients

As previously discussed, soft tissue is not a reliable structure to use for the image merging process. Thus, edentulous patients represent a real challenge. Instead of tooth alignment points, the clinician needs to rely only on radiopaque dots. Additionally, the surgeon has to have information about the gingiva supporting the prosthesis, as this will serve as template base. This demands to address the shape of the prosthesis outer surface (tooth distribution), the prosthesis inner surface (mucosal base), and the notches filled with radiopaque material. As no scanner reproduces both outer and inner surface, two techniques are nowadays more commonly used to solve this issue.

2.3.4.1 Radiopaque Point Alignment

In this technique, either the removable prosthesis used by the patient, a new prosthesis fabricated from a previous wax-up, or a duplicate is used as radiographic template. Previous to CBCT indication, clinician should check for prosthesis/duplicate perfect fit, support, and occlusion. In cases where patient prosthesis is used, the base

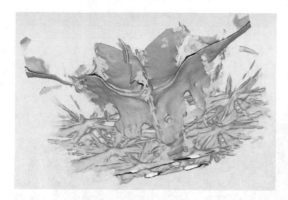

Fig. 2.29 Artifact generated by metallic reference points included in the tomographic template

can be relined under occlusion force to guarantee its position and the reproduction of the underlying mucosa. Thus, once prosthesis is adapted, some notches are performed and filled in with radiopaque material, such as gutta-percha. Metallic indicators are not recommended because of artifact distortion generated by the equipment (Fig. 2.29). Few spots are needed (4 or 5) to be distributed along the restoration. CBCT indication must clearly state that two scans must be performed.

The first CBCT image should include jaw anatomy while using the prosthesis under occlusion. The second, should include only the prosthesis. Thus, patient has to go through only one CBCT while the second is a scan of the prosthesis alone. Two different DICOM files are exported [4].

As DICOM files can gather multiple slices to reconstruct a 3D object, the prosthesis scan be visualized as a tridimensional object (render). Main disadvantage involves low quality surface reconstruction, compared to an STL file coming from a scanner. However, advantages of this procedure are: having a volumetric image of the prosthesis (both inner and outer surface) and having the information of the radiopaque markers, which are the same as the ones appearing in patient CBCT.

Normally, software have a different pathway to follow in order to go into this workflow. Initial job selection should identify the need for a mucosa-supported guide (edentulous patient) to upload the prosthesis CBCT and reproduce it as a

volumetric render; instead of a surface scan. As the CBCT can adjust tissue visualization by determining the HU threshold, a low value is set to visualize the restoration and a high value is set to visualize the radiopaque markers used to compare images (Fig. 2.30). It is important to fabricate precise radiopaque reference points to avoid confusion. Some authors recommend radiopaque lines instead of dots to use the end/beginning of them as reference point.

As supposed, merging process is quite simple, as marker selection is done almost automatically. Finally, once the images are merged together, the inner part of the prosthesis is virtually duplicated to serve as patient oral mucosa (Fig. 2.31). In other words, the portion of the prosthesis that is supported by the mucosa is duplicated to create the surgical template. For that means, correct prosthesis fitting is mandatory.

A few recommendations can be stated as a result of author's experience:

- Prosthesis relining material hardness should be equal or similar to the prosthesis material to be detected as one surface during the rendering. No tissue conditioner material is recommended.
- Prosthesis CBCT should be performed over a specific base, often offered by the tomography equipment. Whenever this polystyrene base is absent, the prosthesis should be separated from the acrylic base with low-density material, such as paper or polystyrene, to improve prosthesis segmentation during the rendering (Fig. 2.32).
- Notches and markers should be neat and shallow. Extended cylindrical markers tend to generate confusion. Round, concise, mid-size holes are preferred. Half sphere performed with a 2-mm bur does the job perfectly.
- Technician can vary radiation dose and distance between slices when imaging the prosthesis to obtain a better render quality. Reducing distance between slices can help delivering a better quality render and will not irradiate the patient.

2.3.4.2 Triple Scan Technique

Despite counting with the double CBCT technique, image quality of the prosthesis render is

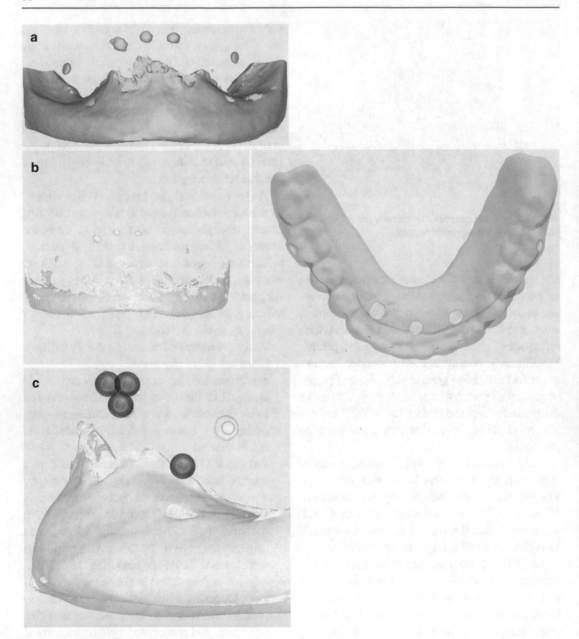

Fig. 2.30 Threshold adjustments help visualize radiopaque dots without scattering (**a**, **b**). Intuitive dot selection is suggested by the software if marks are neat and clear (**c**)

low, affecting the precision of the surgical plan [5]. Therefore, another option is available. It should be addressed again the need to record the shape of the prosthesis outer surface (tooth distribution), inner surface (mucosal base) and notches filled with radiographic material.

To begin with, a stone model of the edentulous area, capable of receiving the prosthesis in correct position, is needed (ideally, a model made out from the prosthesis itself). Some marks are made over the base of the model, far from the prosthetic area (Fig. 2.33). Notches are per-

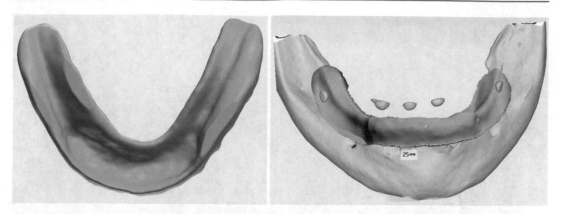

Fig. 2.31 Prosthesis base is duplicated to virtually create the supporting gingiva for the future template

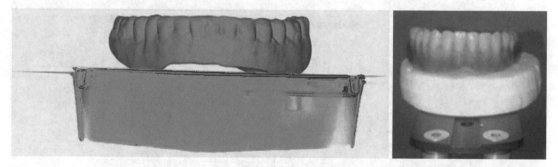

Fig. 2.32 CBCT of a patient prosthesis lying over an acrylic base (left). As both the prosthesis and the base have similar density, segmentation between these two structures is tricky. A radiolucent base is recommended instead (right)

formed in the prosthesis following the indications previously described. Using a scanner, a first scan of the model is done to have information about the mucosa that will serve as template base. A second scan of the prosthesis fitted into the model is performed. Notches should be empty during the scan. Next, notches are filled with radiopaque material and only one CBCT is performed wearing the prosthesis.

The merging process involves superimposing both scans to have the inner and outer surface using the marks present in the model base. Second, the image of the notch present in the STL file is related to the radiopaque dot in the CBCT. Thus, all three files are related and can be used to guide implant position (CBCT and outer surface) and fabricate a muco-supported template (inner surface) (Fig. 2.34).

This technique adds accuracy to the protocol but demands the use of a scanner and more experience on software management.

2.4   Digital Wax-Up

When talking about digital wax-up, two options can be suitable to achieve the desired result, each with its limitations and advantages.

2.4.1   Direct Wax-Up

Implant planning programs provide virtual crowns to be positioned within patient surface scan; some software even allow virtual tooth to be positioned within the CBCT rendering. Most sophisticated software allow the clinician to adjust certain aspects of the tooth, like profile, emergence, cusp height, and occlusal anatomy while more basic software only allow to move, rotate, and vary tooth size.

In general, tooth wax-up is mandatory in modern implantology to achieve a prosthetically driven surgery. This is a necessary step for virtual

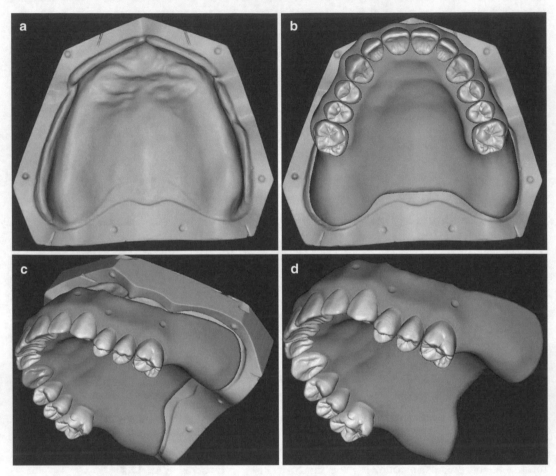

Fig. 2.33 A first scan offers the mucosal surface (**a**) and also includes some marks in the periphery of the model. A second scan (**b**, **c**) offers the relation between prosthesis and model, relating inner and outer surfaces of the restora-tion. In this case, complete denture is designed digitally to be printed and notches are also made digitally to be filled with radiopaque material (**d**)

implant placement, despite the need of fabricating a restoration and disregarding the loading protocol selected. This means that, even when the virtual wax-up does not end with a provisional crown fabrication, the wax-up should take place anyway. Additionally, surgical planning programs cannot deliver restorations. Thus, after finalizing the surgical planning, information of the jaw containing the implant needs to be exported to a CAD (prosthetic) software to select or design an abutment and fabricate the desired restoration. This prosthetic software allows the clinician to determine a margin line, manipulate material thickness, set up material configurations, determine cement gap and other features; guided by the original wax-up done in the implant planning software.

It is important to highlight that both software programs need to be compatible to permit information transferring (see Sect. 2.2.2).

2.4.2 Indirect Wax-Up

As described, virtual wax-up performed in an implant planning software has its limitations. More complex designs should involve a prosthetic software. Moreover, compatibility between these programs is necessary for them to work together. Multiple restoration cases can be challenging if clinical parameters such as tooth anatomy and distribution are altered.

Therefore, some cases require a previous wax-up and a try-in appointment to confirm

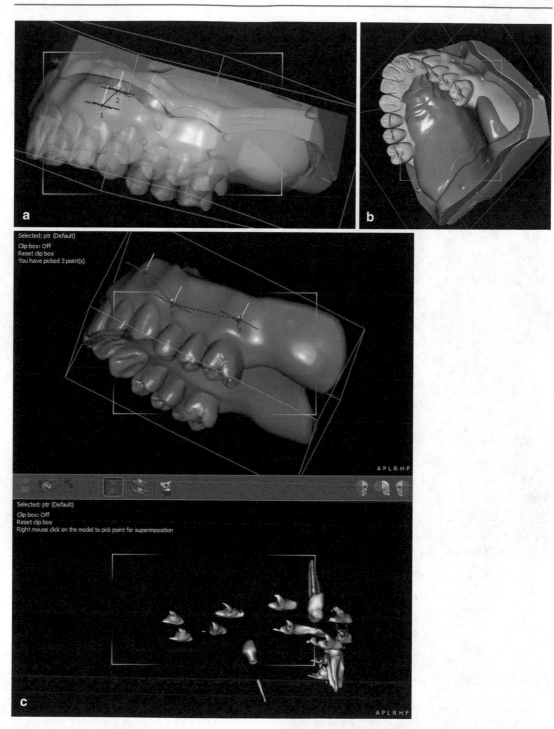

Fig. 2.34 Image superimposition using a surgical planning software relating model, prosthesis, and CBCT (**a–c**)

new clinical parameters and continue with implant planning [5]. For that means, either a virtual or an analog wax-up can be made for the clinician to confirm the prosthodontic plan (mock-up appointment). If the wax-up is done virtually, a cast (Fig. 2.35) or the mock-up itself (Fig. 2.36) can be printed/milled. Afterwards, a surface scan containing informa- tion of the future restoration can be obtained. Virtual tooth library is not necessary if said scan contains all relevant informa- tion. However, if not modifications are neces- sary, the information of the clinical situation is already stored in a digital file; which is the STL file exported to print the mock-up model or mock-up itself. Thus, this STL file can be

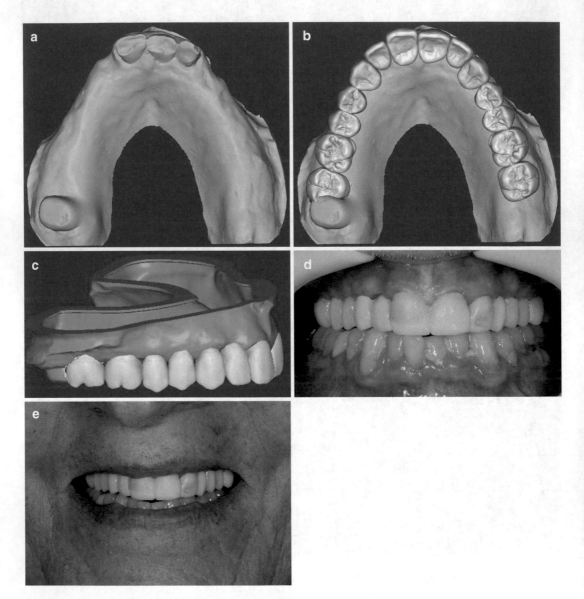

Fig. 2.35 Patient initial situation (**a**) and virtual wax-up (**b**). A model is printed to transfer the desired prosthetic plan to the patient (**c**). Clinical view of the accepted mock-up (**d**, **e**)

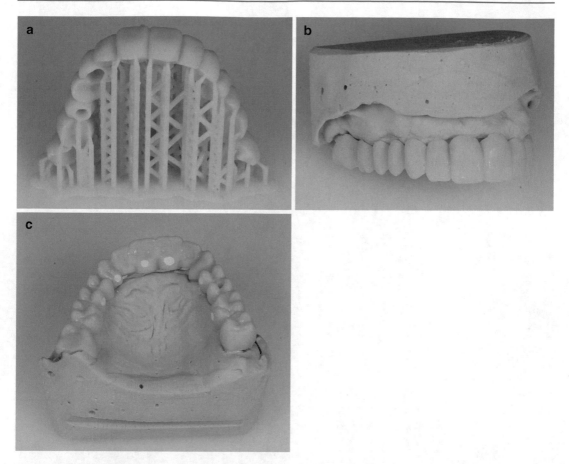

Fig. 2.36 Instead of printing a model, the mock-up itself can be printed (**a, b**). The presence of an already placed implant helps the clinician stabilize the try-in. Radiopaque markers are used to serve as merging references (**c**). If the mock-up is modified, new surface scaninning is needed. On the contrary, if no modifications are made, the STL file created for printing can be used as reference virtual model

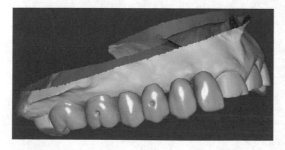

Fig. 2.37 Wax-up of existing teeth is eliminated and notches are performed to be filled in with radiopaque material

uploaded to the implant planning software as the confirmed prosthetic plan.

It is important to match the STL file with the DICOM image; so, the clinician should be aware of the presence of dental structures present in the STL and the DICOM. The mock-up is usually not well recorded in the CBCT image. Therefore, some teeth can be left without wax-up to serve as matching areas for the merging process (Fig. 2.37). Also, if present, extended edentulous areas can carry extra radiopaque points.

References

1. Vercruyssen M, Fortin T, Widmann G, Jacobs R, Quirynen M. Different techniques of static/dynamic guidad implant surgery: modalities and indications. Periodontol 2000. 2014;66(1):214–27.
2. Jung RE, Schneider D, Ganeles J, Wismeijer D, Zwahlen M, Hämmerle CH, Tahmaseb A. Computer technology applications in surgical implant dentistry. A systematic review. Int J Oral Maxillofac Implants. 2009;24(Suppl):92–109.
3. Mora MA, Chenin DL, Arce RM. Software tools and surgical guides in dental-implant-guided surgery. Dent Clin N Am. 2014;58(3):597–626.
4. Vercruyssen M, Laleman I, Jacobs R, Quirynen M. Computer-supported implant planning and guided surgery: a narrative review. Clin Oral Implants Res. 2015;26(Suppl 11):69–76.
5. Oh JH, An XL, Jeong SM, Choi BH. Digital workflow for computer-guided implant surgery in edentulous patients: a case report. J Oral Maxillofac Surg. 2017;75(12):2541–9.

CAM: Computer-Assisted Manufacturing

3

Nicolás A. Rubio and Jorge M. Galante

3.1 Introduction

The manufacturing process represents the procedure used to materialize what has been digitally designed into a tangible object. There are two main ways to achieve this: either by subtractive or additive methods. On one hand, in order to manufacture an object by a subtractive method, a machine has to mill a block using specific burs and rotating axes. This machine is usually the same that the one used to mill dental restorations. On the other hand, to fabricate an object using an additive method, a material has to be deposited and hardened layer by layer. The machines in charge of said procedure are known as 3D printers and material used is usually a polymer.

In general, milling processes tend to be more accurate than additive methods, delivering stronger and more precise objects but also, increasing costs. Objects delivered by 3D printers may vary their accuracy and mechanical properties depending on the printing method and material selection. Costs tend to decrease when using additive methods. Also, clinicians are more likely to possess a chair-side printer rather than a milling machine, as costs, maintenance, and space requirements make these printers affordable and friendly artifacts for general dentistry.

3.2 Subtractive Methods

During subtractive manufacturing methods, an object is created by removing material from a solid block using burs or a variety of cutting tools. As the final outcome comes from the material block, mechanical characteristics of the raw material can be expected to be preserved. Capability to reproduce complex anatomy will depend on the type of milling machine used.

3.2.1 Types of Milling Machines

Computer numerical controlled (CNC) machines are in charge of producing objects by a subtractive method. In dental lab devices, milling process involves a spinning bur that moves in different directions to cut a block that is attached to a baseplate (Fig. 3.1). In contrast, industrial lathes represent a different type of CNC machines; in which the material (usually a cylinder) spins at high speed and the cutting tools do not rotate (Fig. 3.2). This latest method is commonly used to fabricate implants, abutments, and screws, but is not suitable for customized requirements.

Within the milling machine concept described, two types of devices can be distinguished: 3-axes or multi-axes.

N. A. Rubio (✉) · J. M. Galante
Universidad de Buenos Aires,
Ciudad Autónoma de Buenos Aires, Argentina

J. M. Galante, N. A. Rubio (eds.), *Digital Dental Implantology*,
https://doi.org/10.1007/978-3-030-65947-9_3

Fig. 3.1 Milling machine concept. A spinning bur cuts a block that is hold still in a baseplate

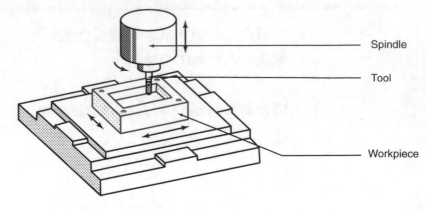

Spindle

Tool

Workpiece

Fig. 3.2 Lathe concept. The material is hold into a spindle and the cutting tool moves without spinning

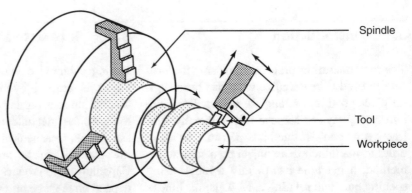

Spindle

Tool

Workpiece

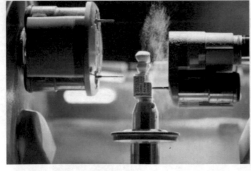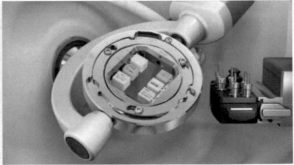

Fig. 3.3 3-Axes milling machine from Sirona Dentsply (Cerec 3®) (left). Only the handpiece can move and so, certain areas cannot be reached. 5 Axes milling machine from Sirona Dentsply (inLab® MC X5®) (right). The material is attached to a moving baseplate, allowing a combination of movements that helps the creation of smooth angles and divergent structures

3.2.1.1 3-Axes Vs. Multi-Axes Machines

Main difference between these two groups consists in the possibility of reproducing complex topography and smooth angles. While 3-axes machines allow movement only in the handpiece, 4/5-axes machines allow movement both in the handpiece containing the bur and the plate holding the material. As its name goes, 3-axis machines provide a cutting tool that moves in 3 linear aspects (left-right, back-forth, and up-down) and therefore, certain areas of the design might be impossible to reach. In contrast, 4/5-axes machines allow all regions from the design to be reached and so, reproduce more detailed and complex objects (Fig. 3.3).

As it can be assumed, costs vary enormously from one type of machine to another. Also, 3-axes machines are usually destined to in-house use, for individual restorations or short bridges containing only one insertion axis. 4/5-axes machines are needed if wanting to fabricate bigger structures, multiple restorations at the same time and/or multiple insertion axes.

For surgical concerns, the machine needed will depend on the extent and complexity of the topography. If wanting to produce a surgical template for a single implant (one drilling hole), the guide can be produced with a 3-axes machine (if supporting anatomy allows one insertion axis to stabilize the guide) (Fig. 3.4). Multiple implant designs will require a more sophisticated milling machine to achieve multiple drilling holes following different directions (Fig. 3.5).

3.2.2 Milling Materials

Despite of the vast offer of dental materials, focus on materials serving for surgical purposes will be made. Most common material used for surgical guides is polymethyl methacrylate (PMMA) for its strength and low cost. This material comes in different shades, as it is mostly used for temporary restorations; but has a transparent option destined for guides or splints (Fig. 3.6).

Another material commonly used for surgical purposes is poly-ether-ether-ketone (PEEK) [1]. This lightweight thermoplastic material has excellent mechanic properties, tolerates sterilization processes and is biocompatible; allowing it to stay in contact with blood or tissue indefinitely while mimicking the stiffness of the bone. Although suitable for templates, this material is usually preferred for implantation (guided bone regeneration), due to its properties [2].

3.3 Additive Methods

Although milling processes offer accuracy and high-quality materials, 95% of templates used in static guided surgery are fabricated with additive methods. This is mainly because of its

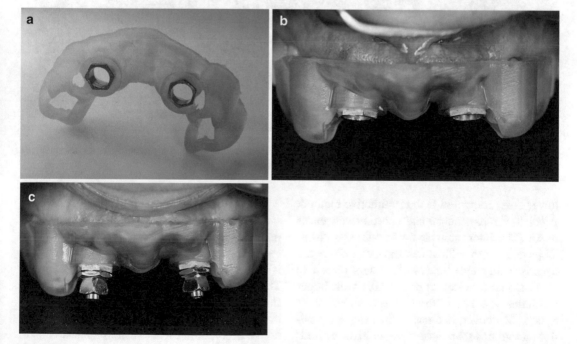

Fig. 3.4 Template for parallel implants with the same insertion axis (**a–c**). Any CAM process can be used to deliver this guide

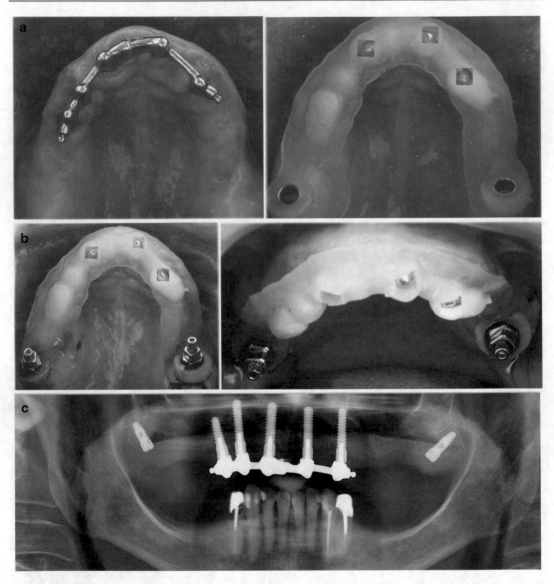

Fig. 3.5 Different insertion axes within the same template (**a–c**). Only multi-axes milling machines or additve methods can be used to obtain this guide

lower cost, compared to the subtractive method. Also, low maintenance and space-effectiveness make 3D printers suitable for in-office purposes. Objects printed with a desktop 3D printer are usually ready overnight while orders placed to professional services or dental labs with larger machines are ready for delivery within 2 to 5 days. Moreover, in terms of final implant position, templates fabricated with additive methods have shown similar accuracy than those manufactured with subtractive methods [3].

Opposite to CNC machining, 3D printers fabricate an object either by material deposition, material fusion or by hardening material layers from a resin deposited in a vat. Once an object is designed, it becomes a blueprint for the software to process it. This model is then sliced into sequential 2-dimensional layers to give the printer instructions to build the object; layer by layer. Additionally, 3D printers do not need "extra tools," such as special burs, to obtain a desired model and both simple and complex forms can be equally achieved.

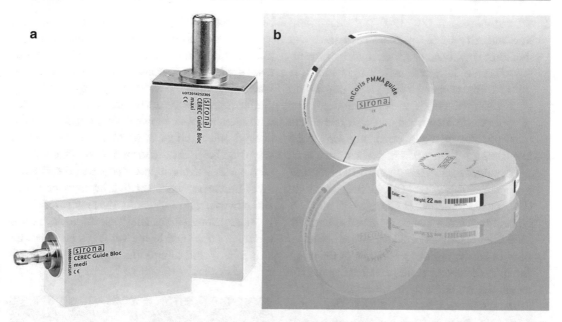

Fig. 3.6 Sirona PMMA transparent blocks for surgical guides, for 3-axes (**a**) and 5-axes milling machines (**b**)

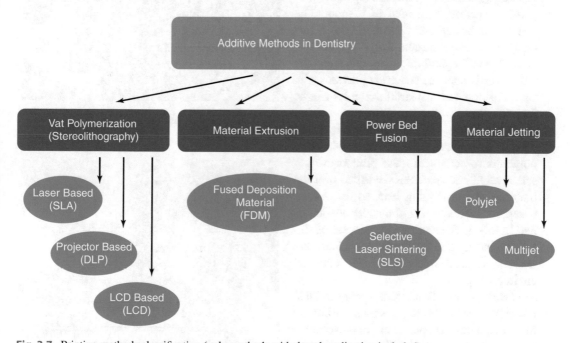

Fig. 3.7 Printing methods classification (only methods with dental application included)

3.3.1   3D Printer Types

A huge variety of 3D printers is available and, as with CNC machining, few of them can be used for dental in-house purposes. Traditional printer classification relies on the printing method used. Also, differentiation between industrial/lab vs. dental office machines has to be made, based on space requirements and potential benefits.

A huge amount of 3D printers exists, as they are used for industrial purposes to manufacture any kind of products. To reduce the specter to the ones that have dental applications, categorization will include 4 groups (Fig. 3.7):

1. *Stereolithography or VAT polymerization*:
   The majority of 3D printers used in dental
   medicine involves polymerization of resin-
   based materials, where an UV light source is
   utilized for curing (solidifying) this liquid
   photopolymer. This is one of the first printing
   processes ever described and also one of the
   most popular methods, especially for private
   use (desktop printers). The light source used
   to polymerize can vary, giving different printing systems: laser light (SLA), projector light
   (DLP) or LCD screen (LCD).
   Stereolithography can be achieved either with
   industrial machines (used for larger volumes)
   or with desktop printers. Because of the printing material used, "resin printers" can also be
   an alternative name for this group.
2. *Material Extrusion or Fused Deposition
   Material*: Similar to a hot-glue gun, these
   machines feed from filament-shaped thermoplastic materials contained in a spool. The
   material is heated and deposited onto a surface by a moving nozzle, where it solidifies.
   Then, the build platform moves down and the
   next layer is deposited over the previous one.
   Both desktop and industrial examples can be
   found.
3. *Powder Bed Fusion or Laser Sintering*: It can
   be used to sinter a variety of materials, from
   polymers to metals. In these printers, a laser
   selectively bonds particles deposited over the
   building platform using heat power. As the
   baseplate moves, layers of powder are deposited in low increments and the process of sintering is repeated. These machines are
   exclusively used in laboratories or industrial
   environments.
4. *Material Jetting*: Similar to a conventional
   inkjet 2D printer, this process uses a printhead
   that dispenses droplets of photosensitive
   acrylic material. This liquid resin is cured by
   an UV light, building the part layer by layer.
   Some jetting printers use laser instead to
   solidify the material.

3.3.1.1 Laser-Based Stereolithography (SLA Printer)

Even though SLA acronym stands for stereolithography, it is often used to represent laser-

based polymerizing. As DLP or LCD printers
also use stereolithography principles, clarifica-
tion on this matter has to be made. SLA apparatuses contain a resin tank with a transparent base
where the liquid resin rests (Fig. 3.8). A building
platform moves vertically through an axis (or
multiple axes) and allows the construction of the
desired object, either in a normal or an inverted
way (Fig. 3.9). The platform moves to the bottom
of the vat, leaving a space equal to the desired
layer thickness, waits for that layer to be cured
and moves to allow space for the next layer.

SLA printers use a single-point laser to cure
the resin contained in the vat. This laser points
at a mirror that directs the light to the coordi-

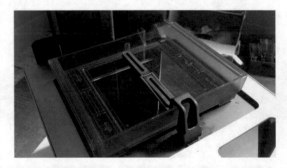

Fig. 3.8 Resin tank for Formlabs Form2® SLA printer

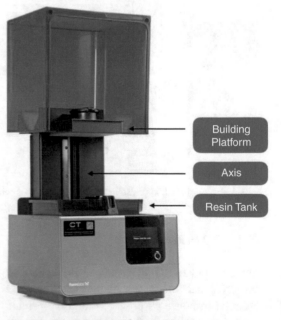

Fig. 3.9 Formlabs Form2® SLA printer

nates indicated by each slice (Fig. 3.10). The beam is delivered consistently to each dot to ensure the size of the light projected in every corner of the slice.

The result is an object with smooth surface (laser is capable of delivering rounded lines) with minimum distortion (light reaches every corner with the same size and intensity). However, the printing process tends to be more time-consuming compared to other resin-based printers.

Layer thickness ranges between 25 and 100 µm. Reducing this parameter results in smoother surface (rounded shape objects) but increases printing time and costs. Desktop printers build the object facing upside down, as the light source comes from below and the platform arises on every increment. This helps manufacturers deliver an affordable equipment but decreases building size possibilities, as gravity force applied to the object being constructed can

cause the print to fail. On the other hand, industrial SLA machines normally use a top-down system to allow massive production without risks of failing or losing accuracy (Fig. 3.11).

3.3.1.2 Digital Light Processing (DLP Printer)

Similar to their SLA counterparts, desktop DLP printers have a building platform which moves vertically and descends into a resin tank (Fig. 3.12). The transparent bottom enables polymerization coming from a digital projector screen beneath, instead of a laser. The whole image of each layer is then projected to the vat using tiny mirrors (Fig. 3.13). Each dot in each layer is cured at the same time; although instead of a dot, a square pixel is materialized. As the number of layers increment, the form delivered is made of small cubes (or voxels), different from the rounded micro-topography that is delivered by the laser projection in SLA printers (Fig. 3.14).

Moreover, as the projection implies curing each slice all at once, printing process tends to be less time-consuming compared to SLA machines (Fig. 3.15). Additionally, as the light projected consists in pixels reflected on multiple mirrors, it can be assumed that these pixels will vary their sizes as the distance travelled by the light projected varies as well. To clarify, the light will be projected perpendicularly to only one part of the vat (usually the center), while the other parts of the tank (edges) will receive a pixel that has some degree of distortion (as it has travelled a longer distance) compared to the one projected perpendicularly. This non-uniform light distribution onto the build plane can influence the outcome, as accuracy is compromised in the edges of the building platform (Fig. 3.16).

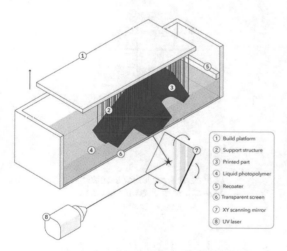

① Build platform
② Support structure
③ Printed part
④ Liquid photopolymer
⑤ Recoater
⑥ Transparent screen
⑦ XY scanning mirror
⑧ UV laser

Fig. 3.10 Representation of the SLA printing method

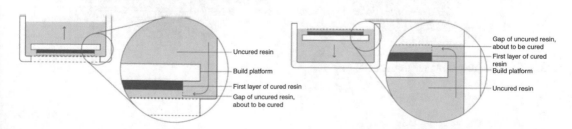

Fig. 3.11 Bottom-up versus top-down printing methods

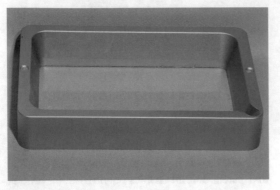

Fig. 3.12 Resin tank for Anycubic Photon® printer

Platform moving vertically (Z-Axis)
Platform
Cured Model
Liquid Resin
Tank
PDMS
UV Lighting
Mirror
Lens
Projector

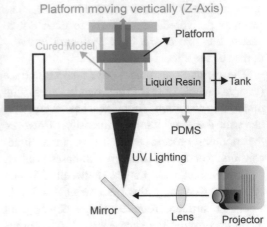

Fig. 3.13 Representation of the DLP printing method

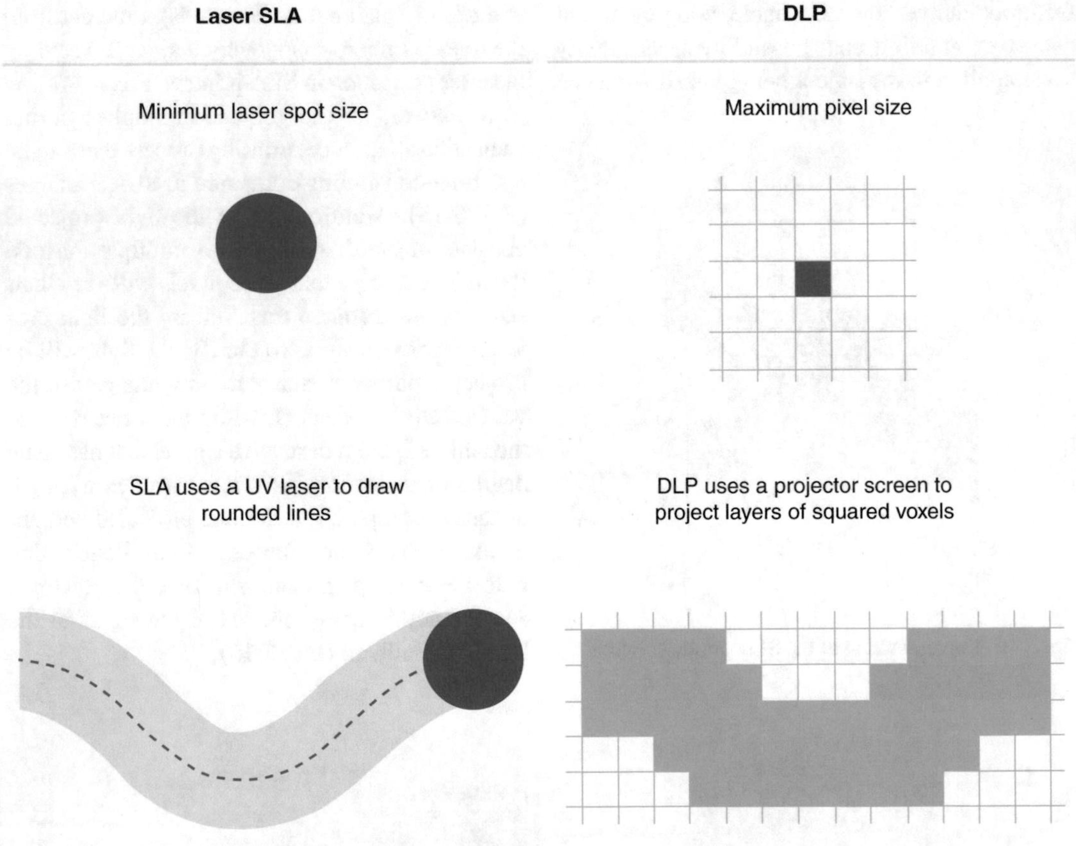

Laser SLA
DLP
Minimum laser spot size
Maximum pixel size
SLA uses a UV laser to draw rounded lines
DLP uses a projector screen to project layers of squared voxels

Fig. 3.14 Laser dot (SLA) versus pixel (DLP)

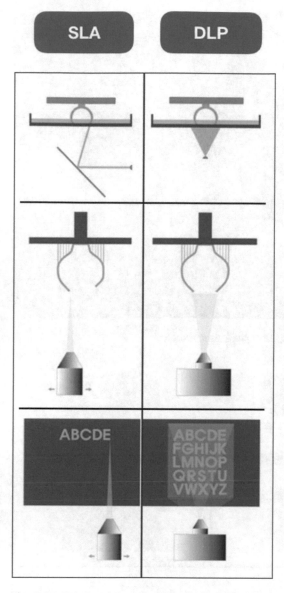

Fig. 3.15 Printing time comparison between SLA and DLP printers

This optical phenomenon can also influence the build volume, as overall projector resolution decreases as build volume increases. Thus, projector resolution needs to be improved for larger scale printings, leading to substantially higher costs. On the contrary, with SLA printers, overall resolution is independent of the build volume; although printing time is substantially increased as the volume of the part increases.

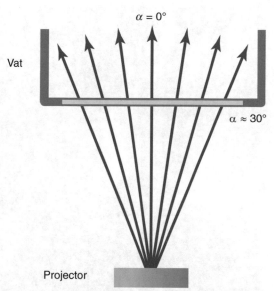

Fig. 3.16 Projection incidence affects pixel/voxel size and light brightness

3.3.1.3 LCD Screen Based (LCD Printer)

LCD printers appeared recently in the market to compete directly with DLP technology. Although still less common than SLA and DLP options, it offers the same main advantage of DLP: increased build speed when compared to SLA. Instead of a projector, this printer uses an array of LEDs as UV light source, shining through an LCD and flashing directly onto the build platform, following a parallel direction (Fig. 3.17). Therefore, no mirror is required to direct the light and so, pixel distortion is enhanced (Fig. 3.18).

A screen acts as a mask, revealing only the pixels necessary for each layer. As the layer is cured all at once, build speed can be compared to DLP printers. As inferred, print quality will depend on pixel density.

In general, LCD printers also use cheaper components, leading to costs reductions and competing with FDM printers.

3.3.1.4 Fused Deposition Material (FDM) Printers

A spool of thermoplastic filament is heated by a nozzle and, thanks to a 3-axes extrusion head, is deposited in predetermined zones, where it cools and solidifies (Fig. 3.19). Then, the build platform

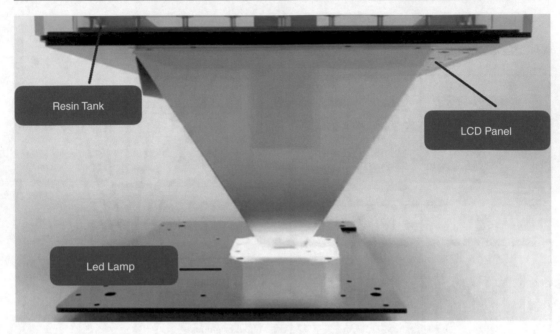

Fig. 3.17 LED lamp as UV light source and LCD panel to select pixel visualization

Fig. 3.18 UV light is directed in a more perpendicular way and no mirror is needed

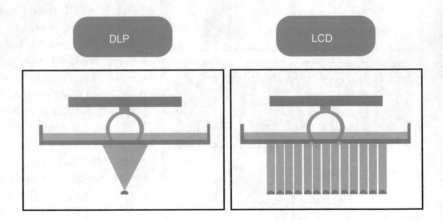

moves and another layer is produced (Fig. 3.20). Adjustment on the layer height defines the speed, cost, and surface characteristics of the printed part.

This is the most widely used technology in private environment, thanks to its low cost and material availability. Additionally, build platforms can vary from a small printer to big industrial machines. On the other hand, FDM has the lowest dimensional accuracy and resolution compared to other 3D printing technologies.

Regarding mechanical properties, as layer adhesion creates weak areas, parts created can be weaker in one direction in relation to others and so, may be unsuitable for critical loading applications (Fig. 3.21).

Post-processing usually involves support removal and surface smoothing. Moreover, warping tends to be a regular and undesirable outcome when using these apparatuses. Cooling process of the material usually leads to dimensional changes and different cooling times (from one layer to another) causes stress which is released by pulling and bending the edges of the printed part (Fig. 3.22).

Sanding and polishing is mandatory after a part is printed, as visible additive lines can be often seen. Cost-effectiveness of FDM printing

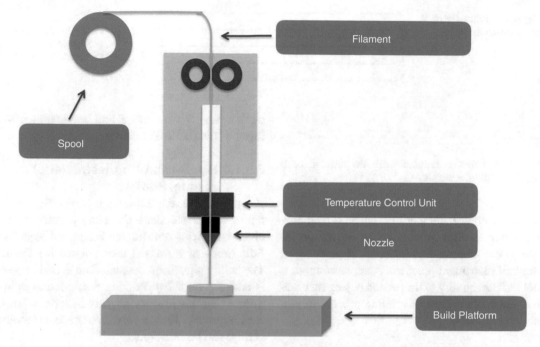

Fig. 3.19 FDM printer diagram

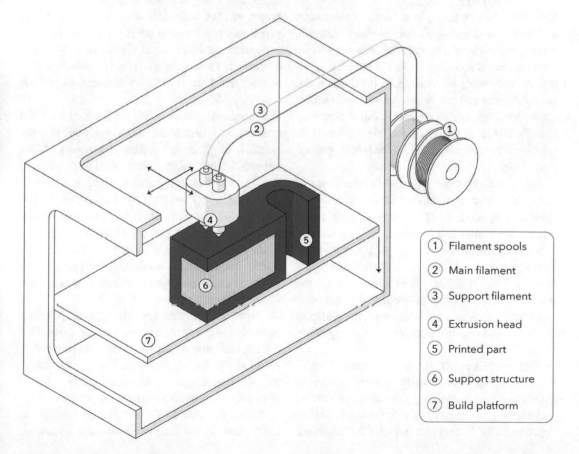

Fig. 3.20 Representation of the FDM printing method

Fig. 3.21 Printed part inner structure (layers)

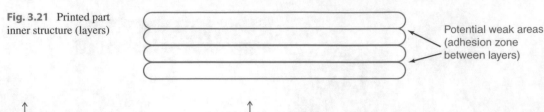

Potential weak areas
(adhesion zone
between layers)

Fig. 3.22 Stress is released when the material cools down, resulting in warping

makes it choice number one whenever productivity comes prior to accuracy or surface definition (i.e., bone models for surgical planning or implant placement practice). Also, as strength is not the best quality of the printed object, mechanical demands make this printing process unsuitable for election.

3.3.1.5 Selective Laser Sintering (SLS) Printers

Selective laser sintering is a powder bed fusion technology and it is applicable to many materials among the industry. Focus in this chapter will be made on metal sintering, as this is the only application concerning dental surgery. Industrial metal printing processes can be also known as Selective Laser Melting (SLM) or Metal Laser Sintering (MLS). Dental applications include, for instance, printing titanium meshes for guided bone regeneration [4, 5].

Laser melting technology uses a laser to selectively fuse or melt metal powder particles. Some printers can produce parts from a single metal while others can produce alloys.

As explained previously, a powder layer contained in an adjacent vat is deposited and leveled using a roller. Then, a laser scans the desired area, melting or fusing the particles together. Once the layer is finished, the platform descends and another powder layer is deposited (Fig. 3.23).

The process needs support structures to minimize warping that usually occurs whenever increasing and decreasing temperatures (fusing and cooling). Post-processing includes detaching support parts (sometimes using CNC technol-

ogy), loose powder removal and heat treatment to improve mechanical properties.

3.3.1.6 PolyJet and Multijet (Material Jetting) Printers

Polyjet and Multijet technologies come from different brands but share the same printing principle. Using tiny nozzles, the head-print deposits little drops of resin and then polymerize them. The building platform descends and another layer is added (Fig. 3.24). Printing resolution is optimum using this process, slightly better than stereolithography. Thus, a very accurate and smooth surface can be delivered.

Due to its multiple printheads, the printer is capable of using different materials; so, different colors or even materials with different physical properties can be used all at once. The result is a combined object, unlike with SLA printers. Moreover, some printers offer the possibility of mixing materials to achieve customized properties (Fig. 3.25).

Definitely, multi-color and multi-material options are the most advantageous characteristics of material jetting processes. Also, extended build volume, increased accuracy and no need for secondary curing make it an excellent printing option for dental purposes (aligners, guides, models, etc.). On the other hand, main disadvantage, compared to SLA printing, is the overall cost. Although industrial and in-house options are available, these printers are more suitable for labs/companies rather than for a dental office.

Support is needed for this type of printing. Nevertheless, this structures can be printed in dissolvable material to facilitate post-processing removal. Some technologies use wax-based materials as support pins in order to enhance removal by using an oven heating process.

Normally, due to the small layer thickness used, parts do not require post-curing. However,

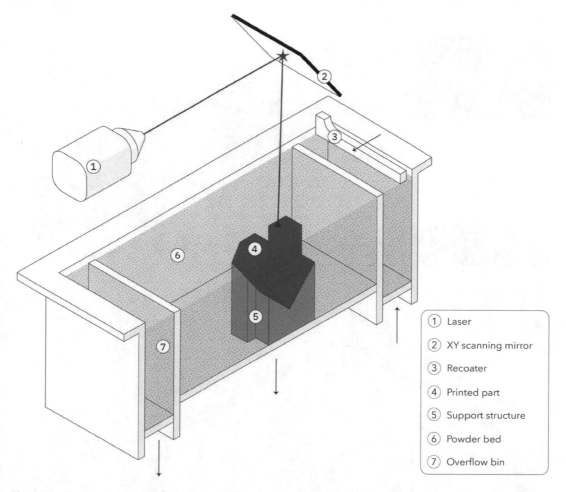

Fig. 3.23 Representation of SLS printing method

post-processing includes support removal and elimination of residual resin.

3.3.2   Printing Material Requirements (For Surgery)

Many materials are suitable for 3D printing; even metals can be printed. A great variety is offered, but not all materials are suitable for clinical use. On one hand, thermoplastic or photosensitive resins can be widely used to fabricate models using SLA or FDM printers, either for bone or for conventional template fabrication. However, specific resins, usually designated with the letters "SG," need to be used to fabricate templates for guided surgery.

Parts fabricated with these resins can be steam sterilized (135 °C) to use them directly into surgery and can maintain contact with oral tissue as they are biocompatible.

3.3.3   Printing Tips

– *Model Preparation*: Hollowed models and resin scape canals are recommended as a way of reducing the total weight of the part (Fig. 3.26). This decreases tension produced by gravity in bottom-up printers and helps save resin material. Additionally, minimum wall thickness is recommended and inspection of meshing errors is highly recommended before printing.

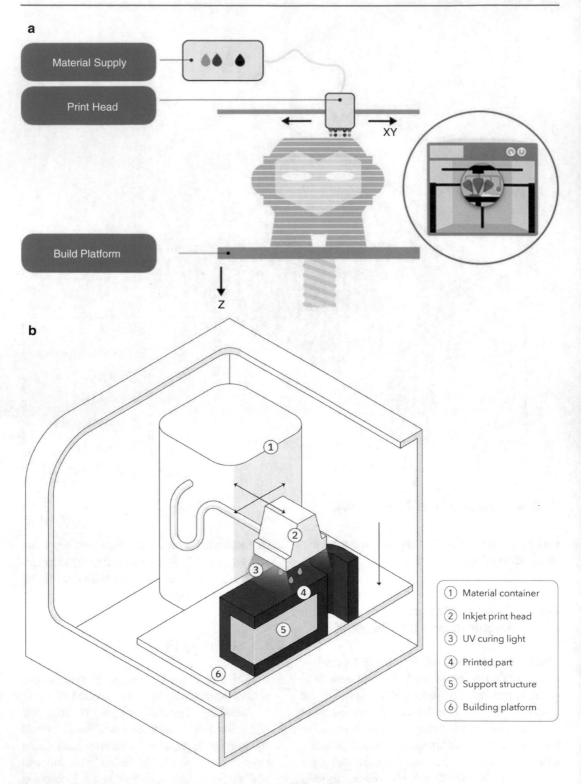

Fig. 3.24 Representations of material jetting printing methods (**a, b**)

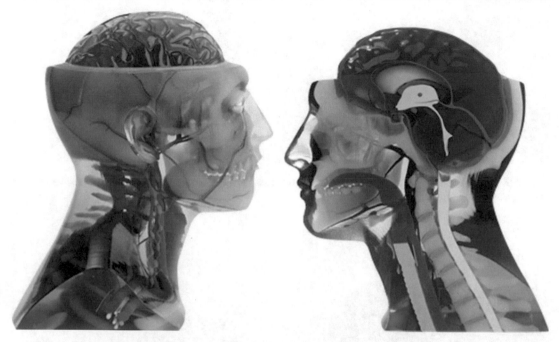

Fig. 3.25 Customized objects can be printed using different colors and/or different materials

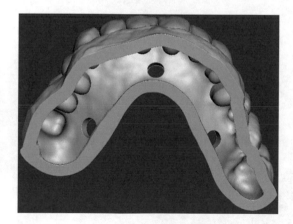

Fig. 3.26 Model preparation to improve printing outcome

– *Support*: Except for some printers, support structure is usually required to achieve a good result. Auto-support option is always recommended as a starting point whitin the printing software (Fig. 3.27). Later, additional pins can be added where necessary and pins compromising critical surfaces can be removed. If auto-support function suggests multiple pins over said critical surfaces, reorientation of the model may be considered. Most of the times,

support structures are printed in the same material as the part and must be manually removed after printing (Fig. 3.28).

– *Orientation*: Changes in orientation can make printing time, amount of material, and accuracy vary. Overhanging parts may need extra support, which may alter its surface because of post-processing maneuvers. Modification on the object orientation can avoid overhanging areas and can protect critical surfaces. Time spent on this step is meaningful if wanting to accurately reproduce what has been designed. Moreover, orientation is more complicated in bottom-up printers, like most of desktop resin printers available. Here, the moment where the build platform arises to give space to the following layer is critical. This step, known as the peeling step, may cause the part to detach from the platform. For this reason, objects should be oriented in an angle, so that the cross-section area of each layer is reduced as minimum as possible. As it can be inferred, support is also increased using an angled orientation (Figs. 3.29 and 3.30).

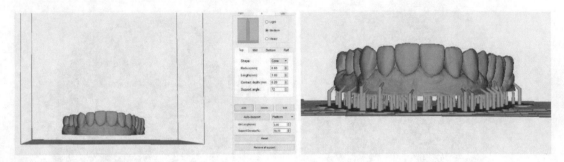

Fig. 3.27 Support options. As starting point, auto-support is always recommended. Critical areas can be preserved by deleting some support or adding more pins

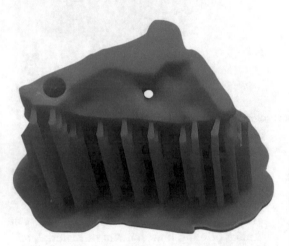

Fig. 3.28 Supporting pins after printing before removal

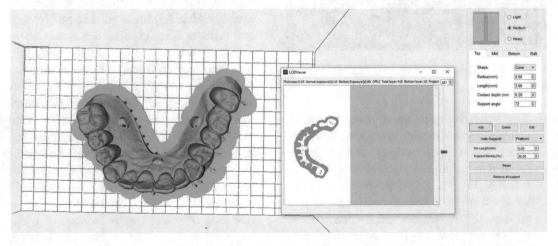

Fig. 3.29 Although horizontal positioning seems to be the most effective way to slice and print this model, peeling effect can provoke material deformation, as the area of each slice is considerable extense

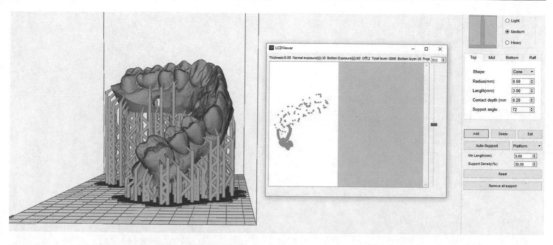

Fig. 3.30 Reorientation of the model helps reduce the area of each slice to minimize the peeling effect. Nevertheless, as height is increased, more slices are needed. So, printing time is also increased

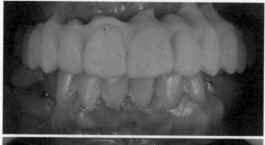

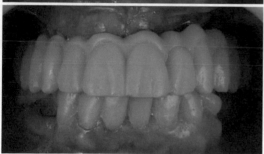

Fig. 3.31 Over-exposed and groovy surface caused by an improper post-processing (up) and correct UV exposure and polishing (down)

– *Post-curing*: To achieve the best mechanical properties, photopolymer parts (SLA printed objects) must be post-cured, either by placing them into a cure box under intense UV light or by leaving the part in the sun. This process improves hardness and temperature resistance of the SLA printed object. Nevertheless, extended exposure to UV light has detrimental effects in physical properties and appearance of the piece. Common consequences are: curling, becoming more brittle, and color changing (Fig. 3.31). To avoid appearance changes, some products offer an acrylic spray coating to use before curing.

References

1. Tahmaseb A, De Clerck R, Wismeijer D. Computer-guided implant placement: 3D planning software, fixed intraoral reference points, and CAD/CAM technology. A case report. Int J Oral Maxillofac Implants. 2009;24(3):541–6.
2. Ortega-Martínez J. Polyetheretherketone (PEEK) as a medical and dental material. A literature review. Med Res Arch. 2017;5(5):1–16.
3. Henprasert P, Dawson DV, El-Kerdani T, Song X, Couso-Queiruga E, Holloway JA. Comparison of the accuracy of implant position using surgical guides fabricated by additive and subtractive techniques. J Prosthodont. 2020;29(6):534–41.
4. Rider P, Kačarević ŽP, Alkildani S, Retnasingh S, Schnettler R, Barbeck M. Additive manufacturing for guided bone regeneration: a perspective for alveolar ridge augmentation. Int J Mol Sci. 2018;19(11):3308.
5. Cerea M, Dolcini GA. Custom-made direct metal laser sintering titanium subperiosteal implants: a retrospective clinical study on 70 patients. Biomed Res Int. 2018;2018:5420391.

Part II

Guided Surgery in Implantology

1.1 History and Evolution of Digital Technology in Implant Surgery

Jorge M. Galante

Since implant therapy appearance, a possibility of giving a solution to a population condemned to suffer has risen. Edentulous patient treatment was implant first indication, by means of a 4 to 5 implant placement protocol in the mental area and a hybrid fixed total dental prosthesis (Swedish Protocol). Consequently, the development of new technologies based on osseointegration principles expanded implant indications to partially edentulous cases and both arches.

First limitations for these treatments were anatomic structures interference, such as the inferior alveolar nerve or the maxillary sinus. Surgical planning was done through X-ray assessment. Analog tomography had almost no application in these treatments, as it was only available for complex medical pathologies. Some implant brands developed acetate templates to superimpose with the images, taking into consideration 15 to 25% magnification resulting from these imaging methods.

Later, multi-slice devices permitted tridimensional reconstruction of the maxilla but showed difficulties for locating major areas of interest, such as mental nerve emergence. As radiation came from a perpendicular direction, some clinicians recommended positioning the jaw in such a way that the image obtained could represent a neat cross section of the maxilla. This was harsh for the patient, as he/she had to remain still in an uncomfortable position during a considerable amount of time (Fig. 1). A complete arch could demand up to 1 h exposure time; costs were high, equipment wear was extreme, and acquired image was not appropriate.

Therefore, moving spiral tomography apparition was fundamental for achieving high quality images, decreasing exposure times, and reducing costs. Thus, together with this hardware, dental software development became very popular by 1990 (Dentascan software). It allowed to obtain cross images every 2 mm and panoramic slices (Fig. 2).

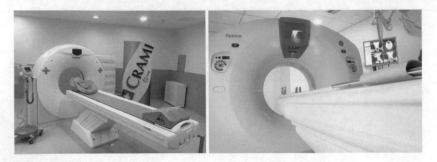

Fig. 1   Multi-slice (left) and spiral tomography (right) devices

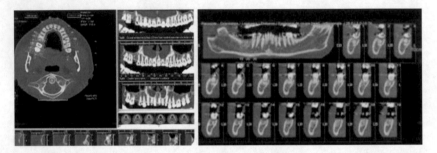

Fig. 2   Dentascan study

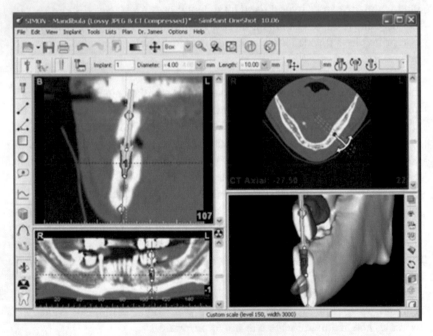

Fig. 3   Simplant software allowing virtual implant planning

Moreover, Simplant software integrated interactive analysis within the program and added the possibility of performing virtual surgery and visualizing implant position in a 3D rendering (Fig. 3).

The next challenge following virtual planning was finding the way to transfer that information to the clinical situation. For that means, radiopaque

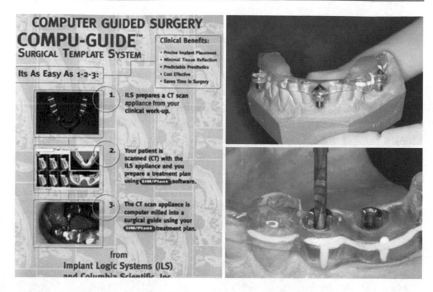

Fig. 4 Implant Logic System (ILS) demonstration and company flyer

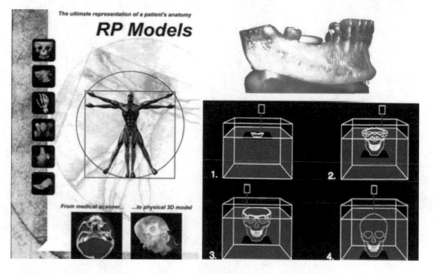

Fig. 5 Materialise stereolithographic model sample and company flyer

templates were fabricated for the patient to use while performing the CT. A company from USA, Implant Logic System, together with Simplant, came up with a metallic device to relate the jaw with the CT (Fig. 4). Thus, the surgeon could plan implant distribution and the company could manufacture a sleeved guide to direct osteotomies. Nevertheless, this was an arduous process to apply for daily procedures.

The Belgian firm Materialise fused with Simplant to create the first template for guided surgery, fabricated with stereolithographic model, using 3D printing methods. This process facilitated overall logistics and opened a new world of possibilities by the obtainment of a bone model directly from DICOM files by a process the company called "rapid prototyping" (Fig. 5).

Finally, CBCT enormously improved image quality and resolution while substantially reducing patient exposure. Nowadays, incorporation of CBCT imaging to treatment and diagnosis is considered a routine. Additionally, the incorporation of surface scan models makes possible to generate a synergistic effect for the application of a wide variety of dental treatments. Among these options, indications for said technology fusion can be: evaluating bone availability, preparing implant templates, planning tissue augmentation by bone block or GBR techniques, creating mucogingival guides, and volumetric assessment of tissue changes in clinical research protocols.

Templates

4

Nicolás A. Rubio, Diego A. Brancato,
and Jorge M. Galante

4.1 Introduction

Different templates can be designed for implant guided surgery. Each type has its own advantages and disadvantages, its indications and limitations. Materials used to fabricate them have already been discussed in Chap. 3, so focus on clinical indications will be made to describe every variant.

A simple way to classify templates is by defining their support: mucosa, bone or tooth supported templates; or even a combination of different variants.

4.2 General Considerations

As explained at the beginning of the book, implant guided surgery is divided into two categories: static and dynamic surgery. The term "static" means that a drill is guided into a specific position to achieve the planned osteotomy, while the term "dynamic" means that real-time drill position is tracked as surgeon manipulates the handpiece, in order to meet a desired surgical plan, [1]. This plan is visualized on a screen as osteotomy is performed, so deviation of the drill can be measured to warn the surgeon. For these means, dynamic surgery uses a sophisticated device to track the handpiece position in relation to patient CBCT (see Chap. 7). Contrary to this, static guided surgery uses a prefabricated template to guide the drill.

It is important to highlight that both dynamic and static guided surgeries rely on previous virtual planning and can transport errors committed during this step. Dynamic surgery does not allow real-time visualization of patient bone anatomy; instead, it offers visualization of the tracking position of the drill. Although this method is often confused with image-guided procedures used in medicine, in which real-time CT or MRI is used to visualize the lesion and surgical instruments, dynamic surgery is based on real-time image superimposition (CBCT and handpiece tracker).

Moreover, the difference between static and dynamic surgery lies on the possibility of modifying the protocol during surgery whenever using dynamic protocols. As it can be assumed, static protocols do not allow modifications: if the planned osteotomy does not meet patient clinical situation, the surgery can no longer continue as a guided protocol and so, template is discarded.

Therefore, data acquisition and virtual planning are critical for achieving a precise result in both protocols. Nevertheless, when using static guided surgery, many variables can influence final accuracy. Relation between template supporting structures and accuracy is one of the most relevant and studied

N. A. Rubio (✉) · J. M. Galante
Universidad de Buenos Aires,
Ciudad Autónoma de Buenos Aires, Argentina

D. A. Brancato
KeepGuide, Buenos Aires, Argentina

© Springer Nature Switzerland AG 2021
J. M. Galante, N. A. Rubio (eds.), *Digital Dental Implantology*,
https://doi.org/10.1007/978-3-030-65947-9_4

variables [2]. Outcome tends to be more precise as more supporting structures avoid template movement or deformation. Thus, considerations will be discussed for different clinical scenarios.

4.3   Tooth-Supported Templates

4.3.1   Specific Considerations

Every patient needing implant treatment is considered a partially edentulous patient. So, template stability can vary depending on the extent of the edentulous ridge or the location of the edentulous area. To be considered tooth-supported, a guide must not present movement or deformation when pressure is applied. Full stability is needed and so, extended edentulous areas or distal extensions can jeopardize template configuration (Fig. 4.1).

Tooth-supported guides are the most precise type of template when analyzing final outcomes,

followed by mucosa-supported guides and leaving bone-supported templates in last place, as the most inaccurate ones [3]. Combined templates try to take advantage of different guide characteristics to enhance accuracy and get the most out of the clinical case. As supposed, retention, stability, and fitting are provided by healthy teeth in these guides. These properties are superior in comparison to other template types.

Fitting is fundamental to achieve the stability that should characterize these elements. Therefore, it can be assumed that template design should be extended to multiple adjacent teeth to avoid any displacement. However, the degree of precision increment as more teeth are involved is questionable. A recent study demonstrated that the number, location, and anatomic morphology of supporting teeth can indeed influence the precision of surgical guides [4]. Recent findings indicate that three posterior teeth or four anterior teeth can deliver an accurate outcome (in vitro

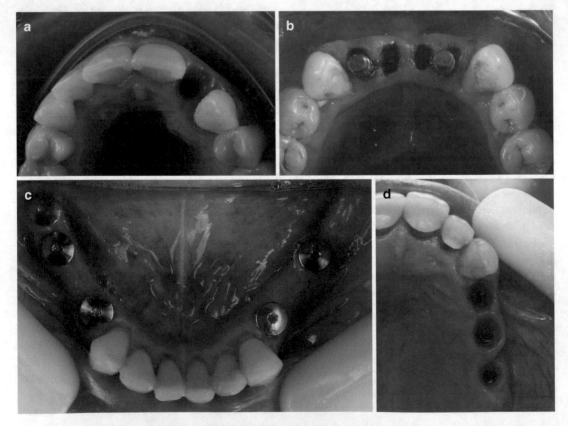

Fig. 4.1 Partially edentulous patients presenting different supporting structures. Although having healthy teeth will surely provide dental retention to the guide, support-ing structures vary among these cases: single implant and narrow edentulous area (**a**), extended edentulous area (**b**), distal extensions with combined mucosal support (**c**, **d**)

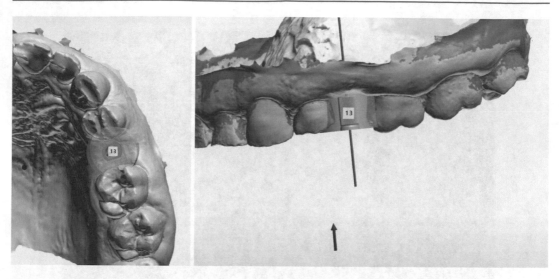

Fig. 4.2 Determination of the insertion axis is done by adjusting the occlusal view (left). Retentive areas are shown with a shadow reference (right). The arrow marks the selected insertion axis (right)

results). Nevertheless, despite the fact that support can be achieved with reduced templates, extending the guide design enhances retention. Then, stability during surgery tends to be more reliable. Reducing material costs and manufacturing time are the only real advantages of using short guides.

4.3.2 Template Design and Manufacturing

As a first step, in every stent that is supported and retained by teeth structures, prosthetic equator has to be stablished. Contrary to the anatomic equator, this is determined by the insertion axis and settles an area where the element can be inserted and removed without being trapped. Said insertion axis is selected within the software by adjusting the occlusal view in order to visualize the area in which the template will adapt (Fig. 4.2).

Once determined, retentive areas are colored or remodeled (depending on the software) to avoid excessive fit. Moreover, retention can be adjusted using software settings and will depend on the CAM method used to deliver the guide and clinician preferences. Some software programs have in-built presets for different CAM methods and different machines brands. Among these options, clinician can find the following settings on template fitting:

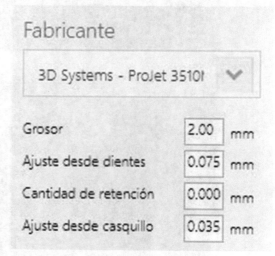

Fig. 4.3 Preset parameters for 3D systems® printer

distance between model and template, material thickness and drilling sleeve adaptation (Fig. 4.3).

Learning curve with these novel methods also includes finding a precise setting for every situation (CAM method and material used, guide support, post-processing considerations, etc.).

Templates designed for single implants can be milled with 3-axes CNC machines, as long as they do not exceed block lengths (Fig. 4.4). Templates designed for multiple implant placement will demand the use of multi-axes CNC machines or 3D printing methods (Fig. 4.5).

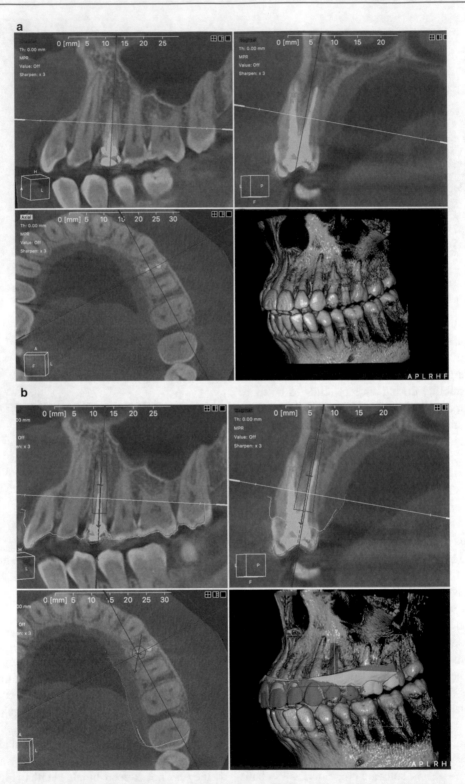

Fig. 4.4 Single implant, tooth-supported, template design. Patient initial situation (**a**) and surface scan merging with virtual implant placement (**b**). In orange, (**c**) a surface model with tooth wax-up is imported (see Indirect wax-up in Chap. 2) together with initial situation scan, in green (**d**). Orange scan will be used to guide implant position in order to meet crown design (indirect wax-up) and green scan will be used to fabricate the template (**e**, **f**). Final design for the tooth-supported template with occlusal windows to assess fitting (**g**)

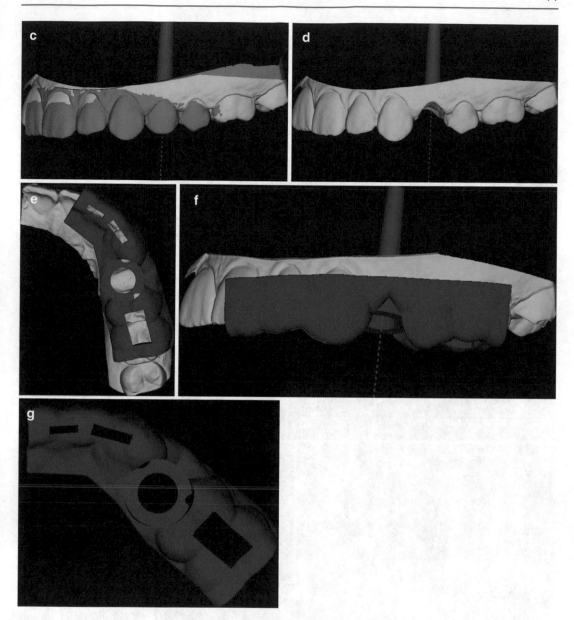

Fig. 4.4 (continued)

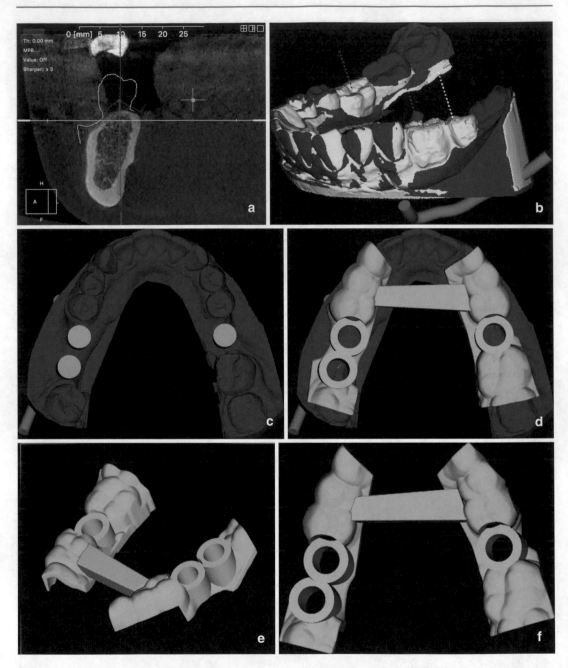

Fig. 4.5 Visualization of the surface scan hint superimposed to the CBCT (**a**). Blue model represents patient situation and yellow model contains information about the wax-up, which helps assess implant distribution (**b**). Once implants are virtually placed, template is designed over the blue model (**c**). Bilateral tooth-supported guides designed with a connecting bar to improve reten-tion. Therefore, pressure applied on one side is compensated by the opposite side (**d–f**). Both templates involve a reduced edentulous ridge which do not compromise tooth support. Patient initial situation (**g**), guide adaptation (**h**), and immediate postoperative situation (**i**). Panoramic X-ray of the implants in place (**j**)

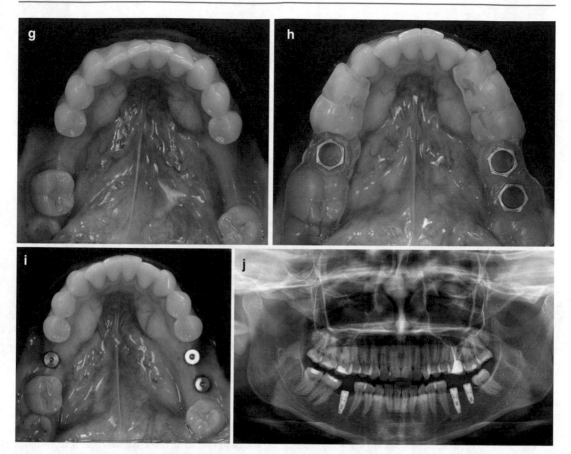

Fig. 4.5 (continued)

4.4 Muco-Supported Templates

4.4.1 Specific Considerations

In these cases, fitting and support is given 100% by mucosa. Retention is absent but can be added by using fixation pins. Patient removable prosthesis must be digitalized by any of the methods described in Chap. 2. This prosthesis digitalization is needed to assess three basic aspects of the design:
- Implant position during virtual planning.
- Duplication of the occlusal aspect to determine template positioning using patient occlusion.
- Duplication of the inner aspect to stablish mucosa topography for template support.

4.4.2 Template Design and Manufacturing

Muco-supported templates can be very accurate as long as clinician is able to address retention and positioning.

First, to achieve retention, fixation pins should be included in the design [5]. Most of them are horizontal, following an apical direction and almost reaching bicortical anchorage. Pins are easily fixed in the anterior region but can be challenging in the posterior zone. For that means, fixation pins can be designed in the palate for maxillary cases (Fig. 4.6). Moreover, some brands offer vertical fixation pins to be used in the posterior region [6]. These are set

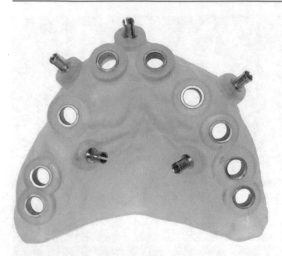

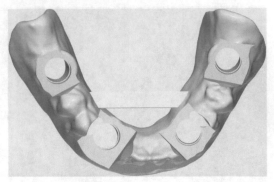

Fig. 4.7 One-piece template with remaining occlusal surface to stabilize the prosthesis under occlusal force

Fig. 4.6 Horizontal fixation pins in the anterior area (3) and additional palatal horizontal pins in the posterior area (2)

within an implant osteotomy, allowing to be later replaced by its placement. That is the reason why they are normally used as a complement to anterior horizontal pins. Vertical pins can be extremely helpful in the mandible, where palate fixation pins are not an option and template support and retention tends to be more challenging.

Second, to meet template ideal position, a bite index is needed [7]. Occlusal aspect of the prosthesis is duplicated within the guide design. Thus, occlusal topography should be as accurate as possible. CBCT scanning of the prosthesis gives poor surface definition when compared to intra-oral or extraoral scannings. This should be taken into account when deciding which data acquisition protocol should be used (see Sect. 2.3, Chap. 2). Additionally, low-quality duplication protocols of patient prosthesis should be avoided (i.e., chair-side self-cured acrylic resin duplication).

Templates for edentulous patients can be designed in three different ways:

- *One-piece template with bite index*: They are usually recommended when few implants are planned and so, sleeves design does not alter significantly the occlusal surface (Fig. 4.7). An exact replica of the prosthesis is done virtually and holes are designed for the sleeves to sit. Thus, if multiple implants are planned, multiple holes will certainly erase most of the

occlusal surface and the template will not be able to stabilize.

- *Two-pieces template with bite index*: Mucosal aspect of the prosthesis is duplicated to give support to the first template and occlusal aspect is duplicated to stabilize the template under occlusal force. Both templates are articulated, as if patient prosthesis is divided in two: mucosa and teeth (Fig. 4.8). This is the most recommended template, as holes for implant drills do not affect tooth anatomy. Guide and bite index are joined together initially to stabilize the template using horizontal fixation pins. Then, bite index is removed and additional vertical pins can be added (Fig. 4.9).

- *Two-pieces template without bite index*: Although this option is available within some software, this is the least accurate template to design for fully edentulous patients. It comprises a first part, which is identical to the gingival part of the previous template and has the holes for the drills. A second part is an exact replica of the prosthesis. This latest serves as a prosthetic conventional guide, as both parts adapt on the mucosa (Fig. 4.10). The problem with this template design is that template positioning and fixation can vary according to mucosa resilience and adaptation. Therefore, this design is only recommended when remaining teeth or implants serve as a reference point to stabilize and fix the guide (combined templates).

Multi-axes CNC machines or 3D printers can be used to obtain these muco-supported templates.

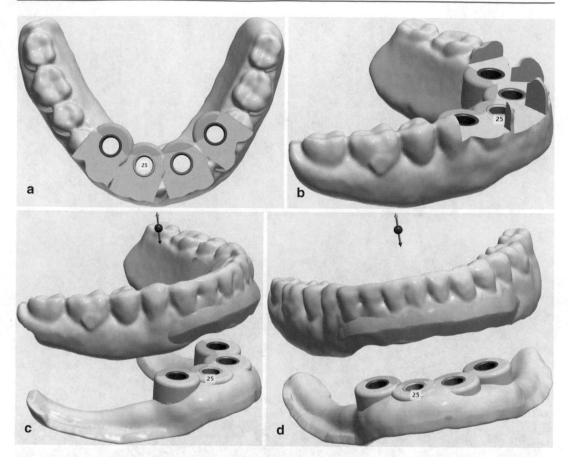

Fig. 4.8 Four implants are planned for an edentulous patient in the mandible. A one-piece design is visualized to demonstrate how multiple implants holes can leave an unstable occlusal surface (**a**, **b**). Instead, a two-pieces template design is recommended to enhance prosthesis stability and template fixation in order to meet the planned position (**c**, **d**)

4.5 Bone-Supported Templates

4.5.1 Specific Considerations

Maybe the first templates ever designed for guided surgery were the ones resting over bone surface, as no double scan was used. CBCT can give all information necessary to plan virtual implants and create a surface reconstruction of the bone for the guide to be created. This process is known as segmentation and involves a tridimensional CBCT rendering using tissue density threshold (see Sect. 1.3.3, Chap. 1). No image merging process nor surface scan are needed. However, careful segmentation proto-col is demanded to obtain perfect fit, as bone topography can be irregular.

As explained in Chap. 1, image merging process (DICOM+STL) helps the clinician get better image quality of the jaws to design perfect fitting templates, as CBCT rendering does not offer appropiate occlusal surface reconstruction. Automatic segmentation depends on bone density threshold determination and can differ from real patient topography, especially in the maxilla. Moreover, customized segmentation is an arduous process. Therefore, these guides have the worst fitting and accuracy, when compared to tooth and muco-supported templates, discouraging its daily use [8].

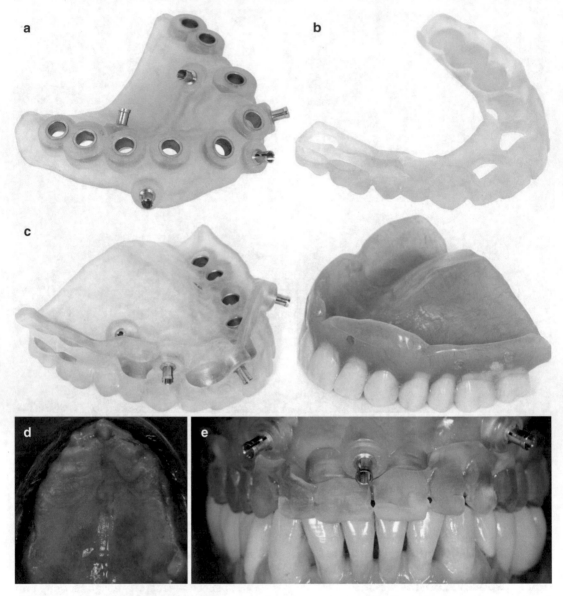

Fig. 4.9 Two-pieces template for an edentulous patient in the maxilla. Surgical guide with metal sleeves, horizontal fixation pins (**a**) and bite index (**b**). The two pieces are articulated showing that, together, represent a replica of the prosthesis (**c**). Patient initial situation (**d**) and template positioning (**e**). Initially, one or two pins are placed to make the tissue punch incision through the sleeves (**f**). Then, tissue is removed and the guide is fully fixed again (**g**). Immediate postoperative situation (**h**)

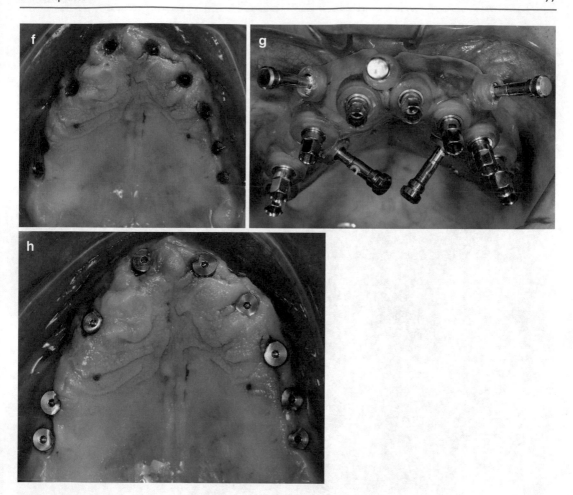

Fig. 4.9 (continued)

Moreover, bone-supported templates promote extended flap raising in order to completely seat the guide. Soft tissue is usually trapped beneath the guide and so, increases misfit. Nowadays, its indication has been reduced to osteotomy guidance in bone block harvesting, sinus wall access, crestal bone splitting or regularization. If necessary, retention can be obtained by fixation pins, as with other templates.

4.5.2 Template Design and Manufacturing

Not all software programs allow template design over bone structure. At least, the process is not immersed in a straightforward pathway. Usually, an STL file needs to be acquired previously from CBCT rendering. So, once density threshold is established, a surface model can be created from the rendering and an STL file can be exported. This STL is then used to design the guide. Customized segmentation delivers more accurate results (Fig. 4.11).

4.6 Combined Templates

Based on mucosal and teeth support characteristics described previously, clinician should adapt every template design to specific case needs. In daily practice, surgeons will come across multiple situations, from tooth-supported guides with extended edentulous ridges jeopardizing their stability, to muco-supported templates needing to gain retention from residual dentition.

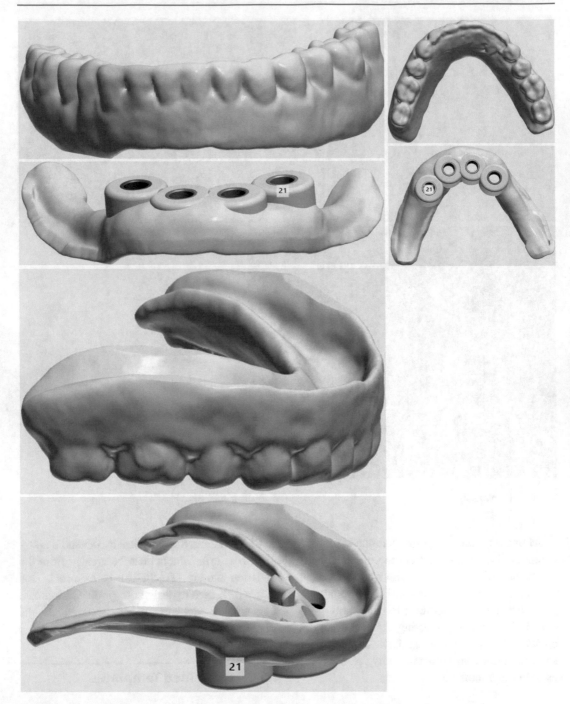

Fig. 4.10 Two-pieces non-articulated template. Both parts have a mucosal adaptation and do not fit together

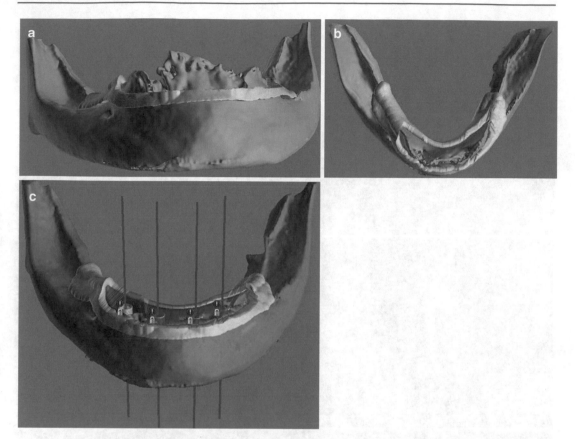

Fig. 4.11 Mandible surface model obtained by 3D manual reconstruction (customized segmentation) and bone reduction guide fabricated with bone support (**a**, **b**). Final representation of the desired bone regularization for ideal implant placement (**c**)

Although a huge variety of combinations is possible, three different scenarios are described.

4.6.1 Tooth-Supported Templates with Extended Edentulous Ridges or Distal Extensions

Support is compromised in these cases as force is applied to the guide when drilling is performed. Moreover, the scenario gets worst if a flap is raised, as template lacks of extra mucosal support. Bending caused by excessive force can even crack the guide (Fig. 4.12). Therefore, adding bar structures to template design is strongly recommended. Bars should ideally connect a distal extension or an edentulous ridge to an opposite area where tooth support is present (Fig. 4.13).

Additionally, retention should be maximized in these cases to compensate any rocking movement or template displacement during surgery. So, more teeth should be included in the design to optimize retention. In cases with extended edentulous ridges and few dental structures available for retention, a fixation pin can be added within the edentulous space (Fig. 4.14).

4.6.2 Muco-Supported Templates with Remaining Dentition

Some edentulous cases are not fully edentulous at the time of treatment. Thus, whenever remaining dentition is present and does not interfere with future implant distribution, template design

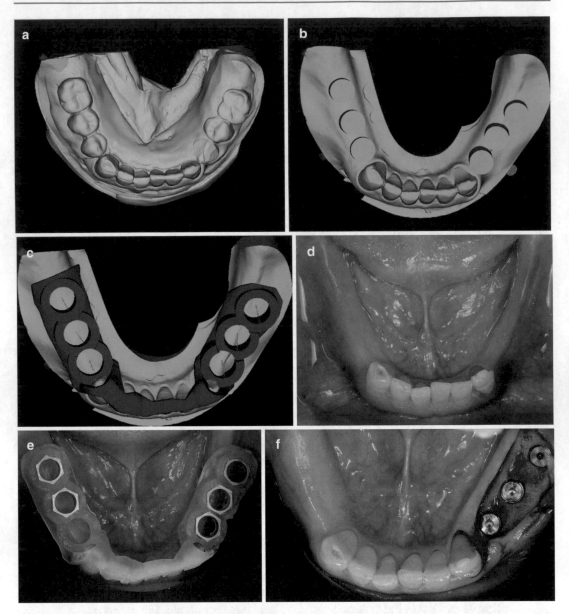

Fig. 4.12 Partially edentulous patient with bilateral distal extensions in the mandible. Wax-up and initial situation models are uploaded and merged with CBCT image (**a**). Template design is performed over patient edentulous ridge model (**b**, **c**). Reinforcement bars are recommended in this case. Patient initial situation (**d**) and guide adaptation (**e**). After soft tissue assessment, a flap is designed in the left quadrant and a flapless approach is planned for the right quadrant (**f**). First, a traditional flap approach is performed to count on mucosal support present in the oppo-site side. Anesthesia is not yet perfused in the right quadrant to avoid tissue swelling and enhance guide adaptation. After implant placement, implant mounts help improve guide stability, as template adaptation in this quadrant is now poor (**g**). Tissue punches (**h**) and a flapless approach is used to place implants in the right quadrant (**i**). Three months postoperative situation, after second stage surgery had been performed in the left quadrant and soft tissue is completely healed (**j**)

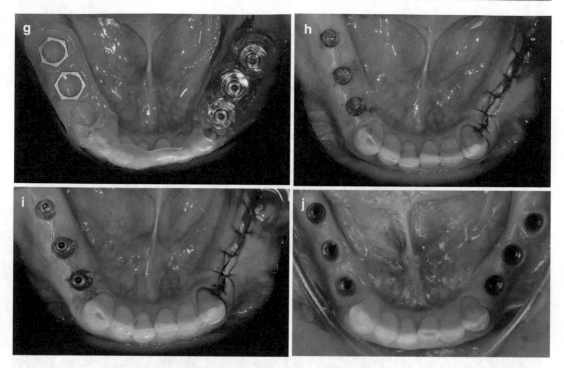

Fig. 4.12 (continued)

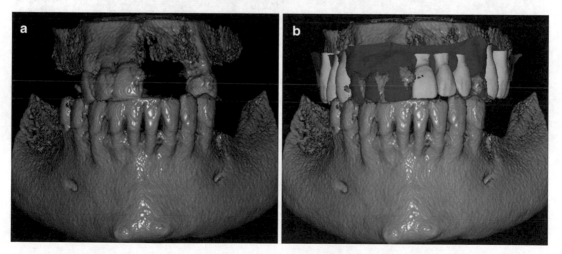

Fig. 4.13 Incomplete template design for extended edentulous ridges. Patient CBCT (**a**) and surface scans superimposition (patient initial situation and indirect wax-up) (**b**). Implant virtual placement (**c**) and guide design (**d**) to obtain a 3D printed template (**e**). Patient initial situation (**f**), guide adaptation (**g**), and final outcome (**h**). Stability in this template can be upgraded by including the palate

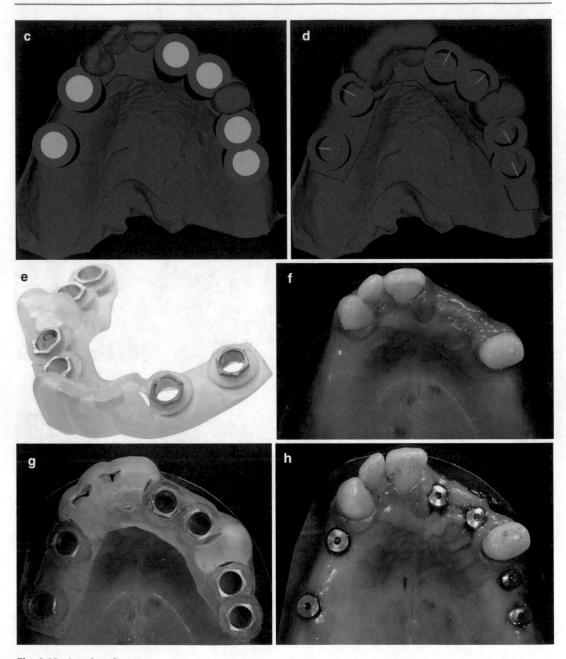

Fig. 4.13 (continued)

can include it to enhance retention and guide positioning. If supporting dentition has favorable distribution, a one-piece template without bite index can be designed, as template can be positioned following teeth insertion axis (Fig. 4.15). If remaining dentition does not allow for correct template positioning, a bite index is necessary

(Fig. 4.16). Moreover, fixation pins can be added to improve retention.

A variable to this technique has been suggested by Ciabattoni et al. [9] whenever wanting to have supporting teeth that are in conflict with future implant placement. In this technique, a first template is designed to seat on strategic

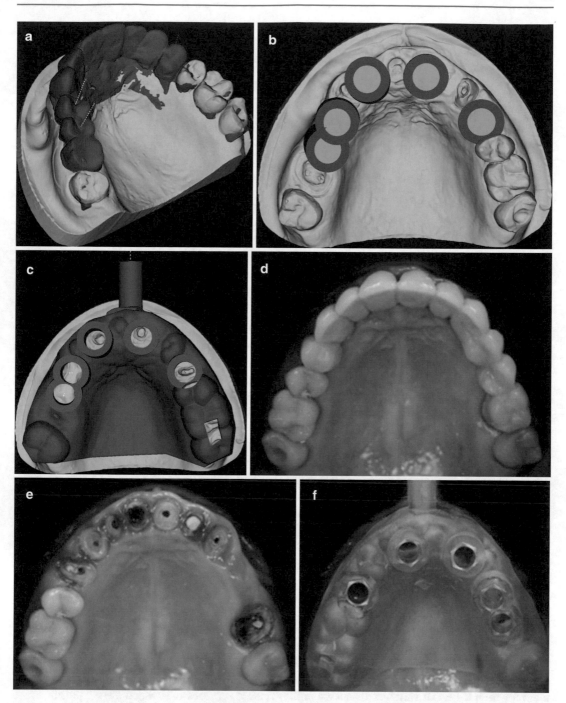

Fig. 4.14 Surgical planning for the partially edentulous maxilla. Wax-up and model containing remaining dentition are used and implants are planned to be driven by the prosthetic plan (**a**). Template is designed over the edentulous model (**b**). Fixation pin is added to improve retention and the palate is included to improve support (**c**). Guide is 3D printed using biocompatible resin (**d**). Patient initial situation (**e, f**), guide adaptation (**g**), and final outcome (**h**)

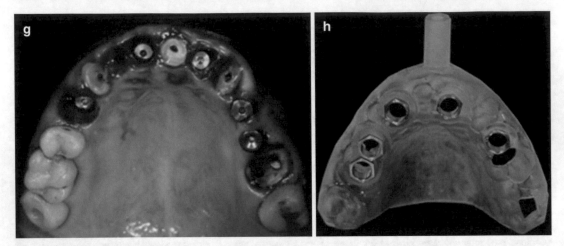

Fig. 4.14 (continued)

remaining teeth and assess first implants osteotomies in previously healed sites (pre-extractive surgical guide). Once initial implants are placed, this guide is removed and extractions are performed. A second template (post-extractive surgical guide) is fixed with anchoring pins designed in the same position as previous pins used in the first guide. Then, expansible template-abutments are screwed to already placed implants and so, new implants can be placed in fresh extraction sockets. Therefore, the first guide uses remaining dentition and the second guide uses recently placed implants to accurately perform the digital planning.

4.6.3 Templates with Bone Fitting

As said before, many template variants can be designed. Nevertheless, understanding the concept of support, fitting, positioning, stability, and retention (which are all interconnected) gives clinician the possibility to design a customized template for each case. All variables discussed until this moment involve template design over one surface scan, disregarding the use of additional scans such as indirect wax-ups.

As technology is usually limitless, experienced virtual designers can get the most out of their designs in order to personalize templates to fit onto multiple scans. Teeth and mucosa come together in the same surface scan, while bone models come from CBCT 3D renderings. Templates can be designed to be supported by dental structures (surface scan obtained by IOS or EOS) and also fit onto an adjacent bone surface (surface obtained by a segmentation process). For that means, both STL files need to be joined (superimposed).

This method can improve fitting of traditional bone-supported guides, as support is given by adjacent teeth and/or mucosa (see Sect. 4.5.2). Additionally, a combined surgery can be achieved with the same template, i.e., implant placement and sinus wall access (Fig. 4.17).

4.7 Mini-Implant Supported Templates

Treatment of the fully edentulous patient is catalogued as complex [10] and so, demands of experienced surgeons following a precise prosthodontic plan. Achieving accuracy with static guided surgery can be challenging. Thus, in cases where no residual dentition is there to help improve template fitting, additional elements can be used to accurately transfer virtual plan to the clinical situation.

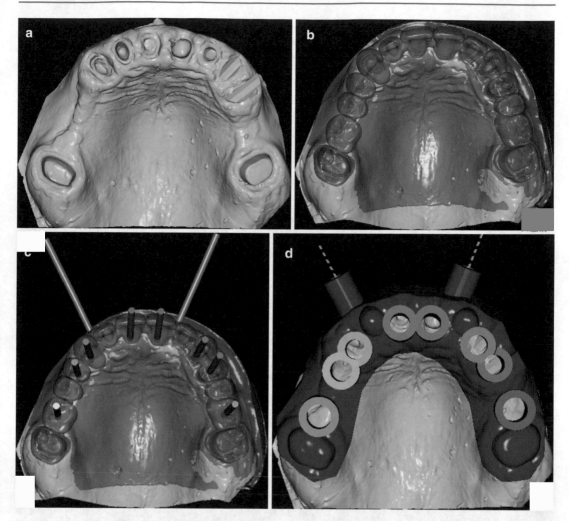

Fig. 4.15 Meticulous implant distribution is assessed to determine whether some teeth can be maintained without interfering with implant placement. Patient initial situation model (**a**) and indirect wax-up (**b**). Implant distribution is guided by wax-up surface scan (**c**) and template rests over initial situation model (**d**). One-piece template is designed as remaining dentition can help guide posi-tioning. However, teeth buildups have low retention capacity. Thus, additional pins are added (**e**, **f**). Patient initial situation (**g**), and template fixation after multiple teeth extractions (**h**). Strategic teeth remain after implant placement (**i**) and serve as pillars for the immediate tem-porary restoration (**j**)

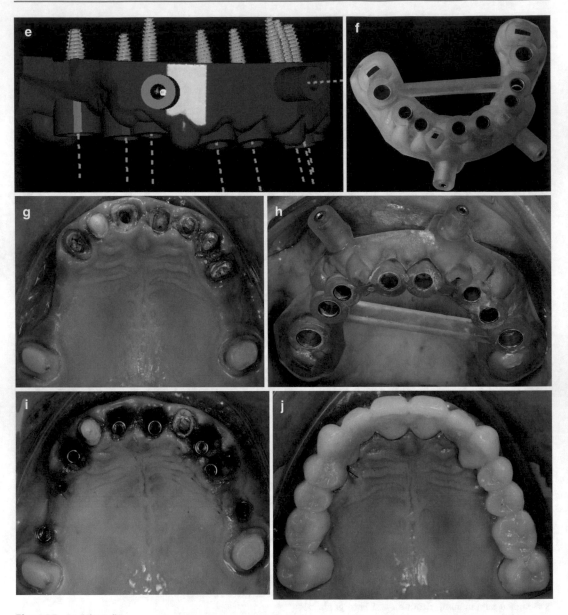

Fig. 4.15 (continued)

Mini-implants, also known as transitional implants, are offered by some brands and can be extremely useful in these situations. Gallucci et al. [11] have described a very precise protocol to approach these cases, which includes the following steps:

- Wax-up try in is performed.
- Mini-implants are placed so not to interfere with future implant placement.
- Template is attached to mini-implants and it is used for CBCT scanning and surface scan digitalization.

- Virtual planning delivers a mini-implant supported template.
- A temporary restoration is fabricated also with mini-implant reference.
- After surgery, immediate implant loading can be performed if conditions for this procedure are fulfilled. Instead, temporary restoration is supported by the mini-implants throughout healing process if an immediate loading protocol is not possible.

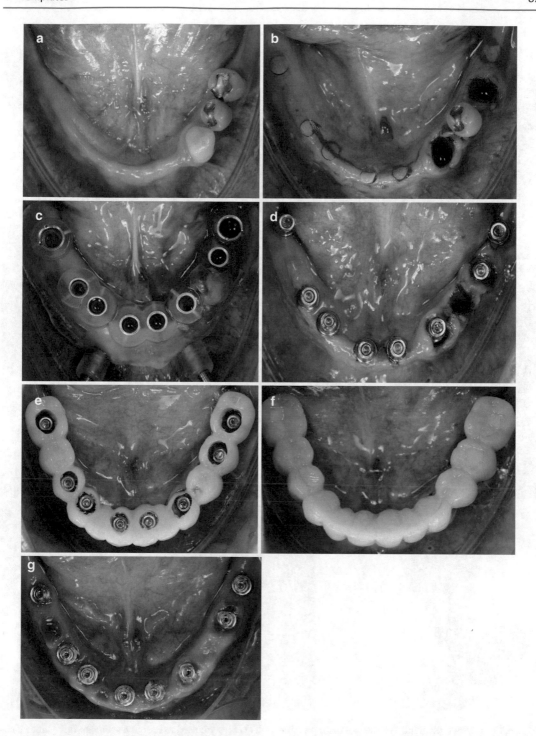

Fig. 4.16 Patient initial situation (**a**) and immediate loading protocol planning transferred to a stone cast (**b**). Tooth number 34 is left to help stabilize the template and tissue punches are performed (**c**). A bite index is utilized to seat and fix the guide, as single dental structure is not enough to define template position. Also, fixation pins are added (**d**). A horizontal bar could have certainly helped minimize deformation during osteotomies, but was not included in the design. Once implants are placed, tooth number 34 is extracted and provisional abutments are screwed (**e**). Immediate provisional restoration is hollowed to permit abutments pick-up (**f**). Postoperative immediate situation (**g**) and 2 months follow-up (**h**)

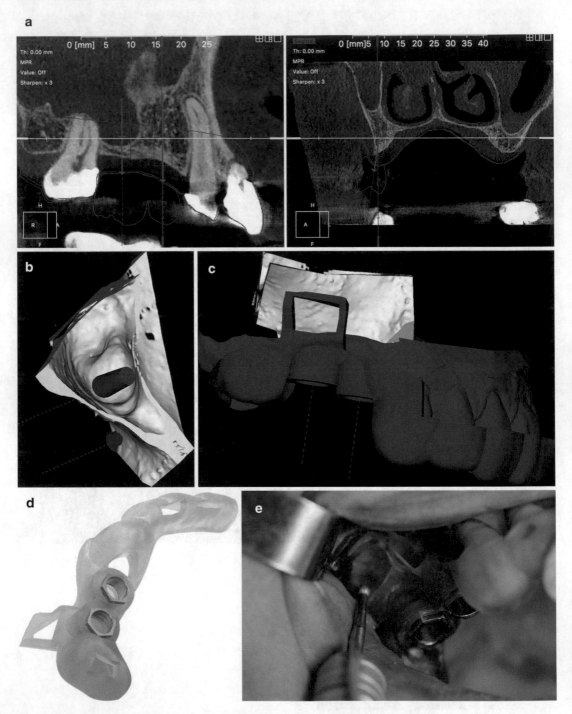

Fig. 4.17 Implant planning for the posterior maxilla. Following wax-up, implant ideal distribution demands simultaneous sinus floor elevation (**a**). A small portion of the maxilla topography is segmented and exported as an STL file. Implant ideal position invades the maxillary sinus as can be seen in the rendering (**b**). Both STL files are used to design a template that guides sinus access osteotomy and simultaneous implant placement (**c**, **d**). Once flap is raised, template is positioned and window delimitation is clearly visualized by the surgeon (**e**). Sinus access from its lateral wall (**f**)

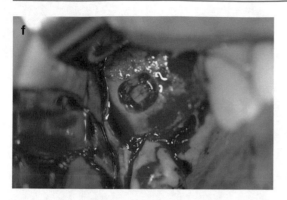

Fig. 4.17 (continued)

References

1. Ciabattoni G, Acocella A, Sacco R. Immediately restored full arch-fixed prosthesis on implants placed in both healed and fresh extraction sockets after computer-planned flapless guided surgery. A 3-year follow-up study. Clin Implant Dent Relat Res. 2017;19(6):997–1008.
2. D'haese J, Ackhurst J, Wismeijer D, De Bruyn H, Tahmaseb A. Current state of the art of computer-guided implant surgery. Periodontol 2000. 2017;73(1): 121–33.
3. Dawson A, Chen S. The SAC classification in implant dentistry. Berlin: Quintessence Publishing; 2003.
4. El Kholy K, Janner S, Buser R, Buser DA. Variables affecting the accuracy of static computer-assisted implant surgery: bridging the gap between clinical success and broad application. Forum Implantologicum. 2019;15(2):102–9.
5. Gallucci GO, Finelle G, Papadimitriou DE, Lee SJ. Innovative approach to computer-guided surgery and fixed provisionalization assisted by screw-retained transitional implants. Int J Oral Maxillofac Implants. 2015;30(2):403–10.
6. Mediavilla Guzman A, Riad Deglow E, Zubizarreta-Macho A, Agustín-Panadero R, Hernández Montero S. Accuracy of computer-aided dynamic navigation compared to computer-aided static navigation for dental implant placement: an in vitro study. J Clin Med. 2019;8(12):2123.
7. Moon SY, Lee KR, Kim SG, Son MK. Clinical problems of computer-guided implant surgery. Maxillofac Plast Reconstr Surg. 2016;38(1):15.
8. Tahmaseb A, Wu V, Wismeijer D, Coucke W, Evans C. The accuracy of static computer-aided implant surgery: a systematic review and meta-analysis. Clin Oral Implants Res. 2018;29(Suppl 16):416–35.
9. Tahmaseb A, Wu V, Wismeijer D, Coucke W, Evans C. The accuracy of static computer-aided implant surgery: a systematic review and meta- analysis. Clin Oral Implants Res. 2018;29(Suppl 16):416–35.
10. Verhamme LM, Meijer GJ, Bergé SJ, Soehardi RA, Xi T, de Haan AF, Maal TJ. An accuracy study of computer-planned implant placement in the augmented maxilla using mucosa-supported surgical templates. Clin Implant Dent Relat Res. 2014;17(6):1154–63.
11. Verhamme LM, Meijer GJ, Boumans T, de Haan AF, Bergé SJ, Maal TJ. A clinically relevant accuracy study of computer-planned implant placement in the edentulous maxilla using mucosa-supported surgical templates. Clin Implant Dent Relat Res. 2015;17(2):343–52.

Implant Drilling Systems

5

Diego A. Brancato, Jorge M. Galante,
and Nicolás A. Rubio

5.1 Introduction

Until this point in the textbook, only software considerations have been described in order to understand the surgical planning workflow. However, implantology has countless options regarding hardware as well. As with traditional implant surgery, implant and instrument selection can influence the outcome. Overall precision depends on data acquisition variables (CAI), adequate template design (CAD), proper manufacturing (CAM) and, of course, optimal surgical performance.

Clinical experience is decisive to achieve predictable outcomes; and predictable outcomes is what guided surgery aims for. Operator expertise has been described as a requirement for both traditional and guided implant surgery success [1]. Disregarding this factor, which demands a learning curve that is certainly different among clinicians, surgical instruments have to be also contemplated.

Even more critical than when performing traditional implant placement, guided surgery demands that each implant system has its own specific drilling protocol. This includes not

D. A. Brancato (✉)
KeepGuide, Buenos Aires, Argentina

J. M. Galante · N. A. Rubio
Universidad de Buenos Aires,
Ciudad Autónoma de Buenos Aires, Argentina

only drills, but also sleeves, handles, drivers, pins, and virtual libraries compatible with the selected CAD method. Therefore, not all implant systems are compatible with guided surgery; neither one implant system alone addresses all guided surgery needs.

Regarding the surgical phase, the first variable influencing accuracy certainly depends on the drilling system used, as templates can be used with different drilling protocols. These options are discussed in this chapter.

The second variable includes different implant placement techniques using guided surgery and/or any combination of tools available within the protocols (i.e., guided drilling and free-handed implant placement versus fully guided protocols). These latest options will be attended on the following chapter.

5.2 General Considerations

To analyze available options among all implant systems, five categories of drilling instruments are described. Templates made from virtual planning, but not containing a restrictive hole to guide the drills, are not be taken into account; as they are not part of the static guided surgery (s-CAIS) protocols. In relation to this, the term "static" refers to the restriction of drill lateral movements or angulation changes during osteotomy preparations.

© Springer Nature Switzerland AG 2021
J. M. Galante, N. A. Rubio (eds.), *Digital Dental Implantology*,
https://doi.org/10.1007/978-3-030-65947-9_5

Implant guided systems (surgical kits) can be divided into two groups: the ones that offer guided segments included within the drills and the ones that offer handle tools to adapt each drill to the sleeve hole. Both of them provide their metal sleeves to be attached into the guide. Moreover, templates can be fabricated to hold this metal sleeve or designed with the sleeve incorporated in the material.

Tolerance between objects is described as a permissible limit of a physical distance or space for these objects to fit or function. This is a critical aspect of overall precision in guided surgery as different tolerances between drilling systems have a direct impact on drilling accuracy [2]. As assumed, the sum of instruments needed to perform the osteotomy increases tolerance and so, influence accuracy.

5.3   Sleeved Surgical Guides

Templates are designed with their corresponding drilling hole to receive a metal sleeve, provided by each implant brand. The clinician may find either systems with multiple sleeve options for different implant diameters (or mesio-distal spaces), or systems that offer a single sleeve model to fit all necessities (Figs. 5.1, 5.2, and 5.3). Guide design contemplates gap (tolerance) between hole and sleeve. As explained in the previous chapter, software settings of this gap depend on the CAM process and material selected; as well as manufacturer experience in CAM processing and post-processing.

As assumed, the gap should be as narrow as possible to minimize inaccuracies caused by sleeve displacement [3]. Metal sleeves must be

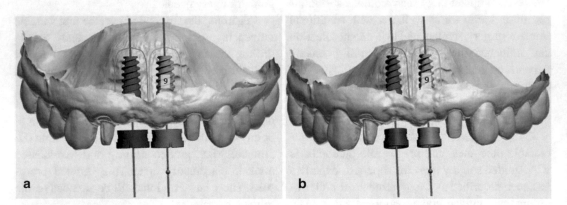

Fig. 5.1 Different sleeves are offered for different implant diameters (or even different mesio-distal spaces) within the same implant company

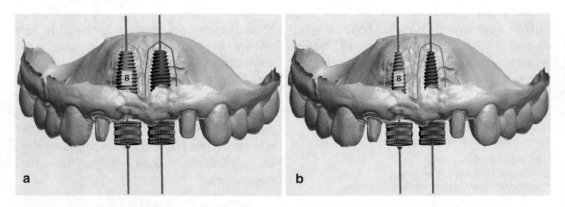

Fig. 5.2 Same sleeve option is presented for narrow and regular implants within the same implant company

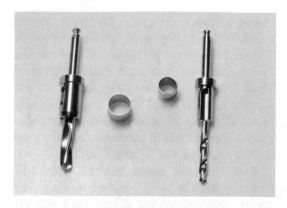

Fig. 5.3 Different sleeves together with their different guided drills, for either regular or narrow platform implants

fixed to the template with fluid resin. Some software allow to design a tiny channel for the clinician to inject this fluid resin once the sleeved is positioned (Fig. 5.4).

These types of guides (sleeved) are the most common ones and can be fabricated either with subtractive or additive methods. One of the most critical aspects when performing a guided osteotomy is tolerance between drill and hole. As stated before, drilling instruments and sleeves are both fabricated and delivered by implant companies. Thus, precision in surgical instrument fabrication by each brand has to be taken into account when selecting an implant system for

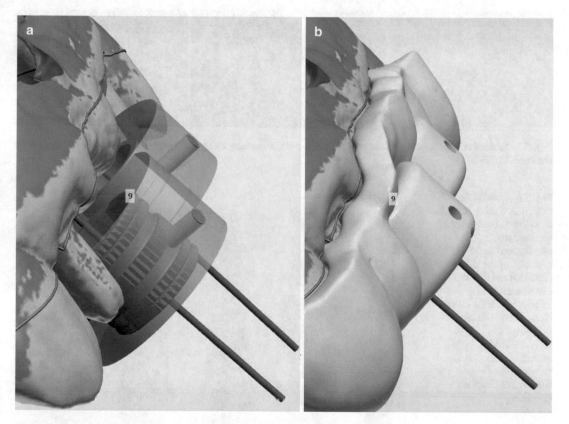

Fig. 5.4 Design of channels for sleeve adhesion to the guide by means of fluid resin

guided surgery. This is the same scenario as traditional implant surgery: tolerance within product manufacturing is one of the keys of every implant system precision.

Two types of instruments fit on the sleeve: a drill or a handle, depending on the system used (Fig. 5.5).

5.3.1 GUIDED DRILL Systems (for Sleeved Surgical Guides)

The metal sleeve in these systems receives a drill with special characteristics, as it has a cutting segment and a guided segment (Fig. 5.6). The cutting portion is designed following traditional spiraled drills, in sequential diameter and length. The guided segment is represented by a cylinder that fits into the sleeve and guides osteotomy. While the cutting portion varies, the guided part remains identical for all drills. Accessory instruments such as punches and drivers also contain a guided segment which corresponds to the inner diameter of the metal sleeve (Fig. 5.7).

Each implant length has its own drill. Nevertheless, it is strongly recommended to use a stepped protocol to reach the desired length [4], taking into account that the guided segment of the drill should be always positioned within the sleeve before cutting. At least, half of the guided

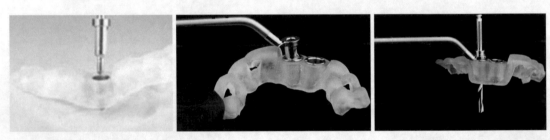

Fig. 5.5 Guided drill fitting into the sleeve (left) and handle fitting into the sleeve (center). Drill diameter is adapted by the handle (right)

Fig. 5.6 Guided drills design. A cutting portion is followed by a guided segment that corresponds to the inner diameter of the sleeve. Note that the first three drills contain information for a smaller sleeve while the other two adapt to a bigger diameter sleeve, indicating this system has different sleeve sizes for different implant diameters

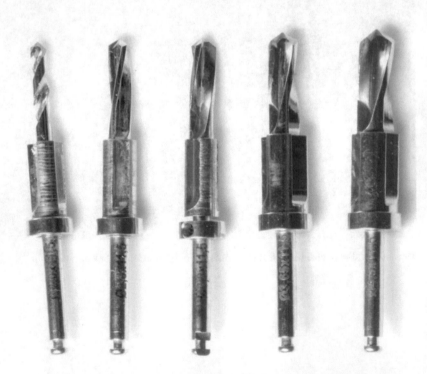

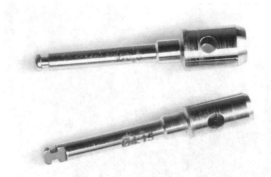

Fig. 5.7 Accessory instruments with guided segment (tissue punches)

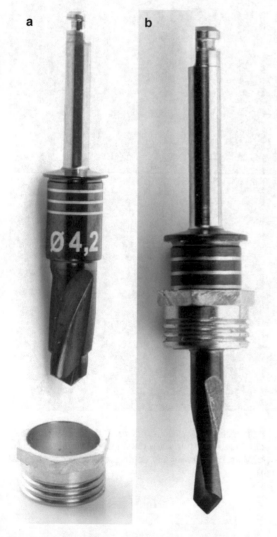

Fig. 5.8 Guided drills with their cutting and guided segments. Half the length of the guided segment must be positioned within the sleeve for the drill to be guided. Therefore, a stepped approach is recommended, starting with initial lengths until reaching desired final depth

part should be inside the sleeve before starting drilling (Fig. 5.8). To give an example: if wanting to achieve an osteotomy for a 12 mm length implant, drilling should be sequenced (8 mm–10 mm–12 mm) in every instrument used. Moreover, in order to help with overall guidance protocol, all systems include a cortical drill, often very short, to permit a smooth preparation.

An inconvenience, usually seen when using this system, is running into an obstacle that avoids reaching the desired depth. This is because most of the systems use an active portion equal to the implant length, immediately followed by the guided segment, which is considerably wider. Thus, this segment can run into soft or hard tissues at the cortical level (Fig. 5.9). This problem is registered whenever not removing the tissue punch correctly, whenever pinching the flap, whenever having an irregular bone surface and whenever planning sub-crestal preparations. To solve this issue, meticulous tissue punch removal (flapless surgeries) and soft tissue separation is recommended. Additionally, sub-crestal preparations may need to use the following length drills to reach the desired depth; or use profile drills to eliminate the stop (Fig. 5.10).

A potential solution to this issue is adding a non-cutting segment to the drills, between guided and cutting parts. This issue is not only visualized when drilling, but also when placing the implant. Some implant mounts have slim designs and so, do not interfere with sub-crestal placement. Others instead, have mounts wider than the implant shoulder and so, can hinder sub-crestal implant placement, especially in flapless surgery where bone topography is hidden from sight (Fig. 5.11).

In guided drill systems, distance between implant shoulder and sleeve position, known as offset, tends to be the same for all planned implants. This is because said offset is already stablished in every instrument of the surgical cassette. Main disadvantage of this fixed distance is the impossibility to customize it in different clinical situations. On the contrary, a clear advantage of uniform offset is that the implant driver has a clear stop that indicates that implant has reached the desired depth (Fig. 5.12). This is especially advantageous in posterior areas where visualization is often compromised.

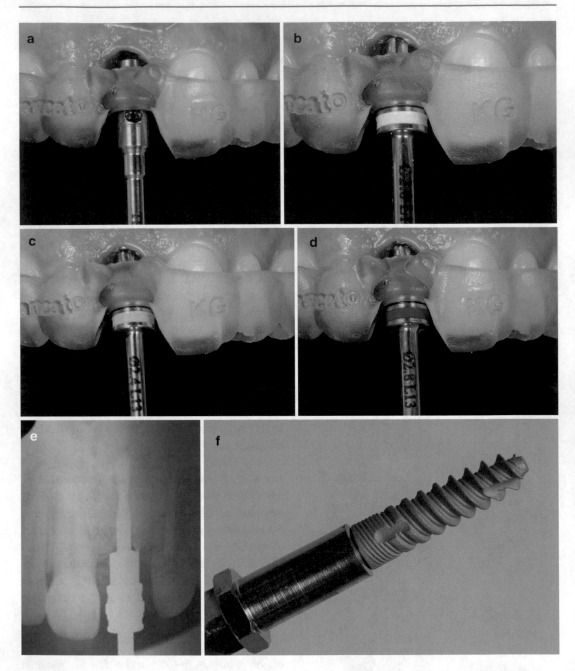

Fig. 5.9 Single implant case with a guided drill system, from AlphaBioTec®. A tissue punch is performed to eliminate all possible soft tissue interference (**a**), followed by a stepped protocol with drill diameter increments (**b–d**). Crestal bone interference can be seen at the rx (**e**), so, slight profile adjustment needs to be done. Note the horizontal platform shift when the implant is mounted on the guided driver (**f**). Implant depth position is corroborated (**g**)

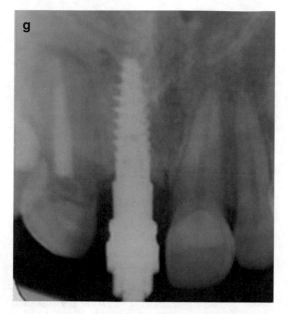

Fig. 5.9 (continued)

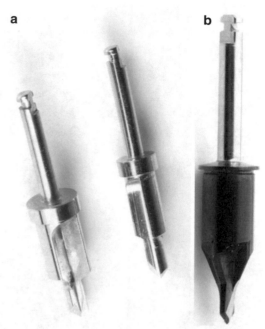

Fig. 5.10 Cortical drills for initial bed preparation

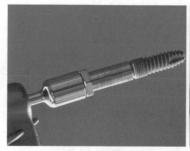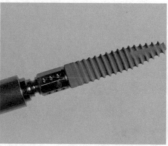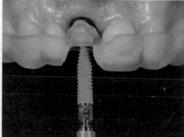

Fig. 5.11 Implant driver wider than implant platform (left), implant driver with switch platform (center and right)

To summarize, special considerations must be taken into account when planning deep implant placement procedures. On the other hand, guided drill systems tend to simplify osteotomy protocols and reduce gaps and tolerance accumulations, compared to the following systems described [5].

5.3.2 DRILL HANDLE Systems (for Sleeved Surgical Guides)

Metal sleeves in these systems receive a handle that reduces the master cylinder diameter into a smaller one that receives the drill, similarly to a reducing key (Figs. 5.13 and 5.14). Drills have

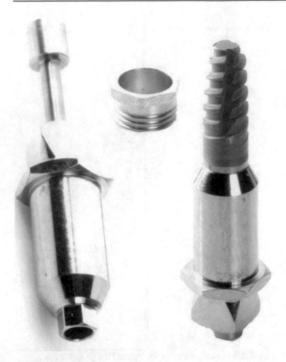

Fig. 5.12 Implant driver with guided segment and visual depth stop

the same design as conventional ones but have a stop at the coronal level that meets the handle when reaching the desired depth. As these drills maintain the same diameter along the instrument, sub-crestal preparation is not an issue. Tissue interference is not usually a problem with this system; however, implant driver usually has the sleeve diameter and can suffer the same pitfalls described previously for deep implant positioning.

Drill is fully guided during the whole process, as it goes through the handle. Thus, only one drill of each diameter can be used without the need of a stepped protocol. Normally, these systems offer variable offsets to customize every clinical situation, even within the same patient. To achieve this, different handle heights and drill lengths are also available to allow for distance compensation [4] (Figs. 5.15 and 5.16).

A more complex scenario is presented to the clinician with these systems, compared to the guided drill systems. Manipulation of several variables includes being aware of sleeve offset,

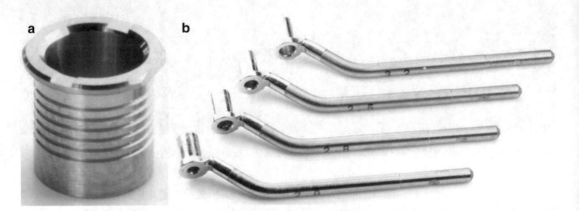

Fig. 5.13 Master sleeve and reducing keys that adapt and modify the inner diameter of the drilling hole

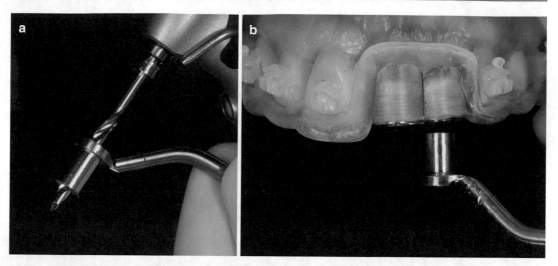

Fig. 5.14 Adapting key allows smaller drills fit into the sleeve

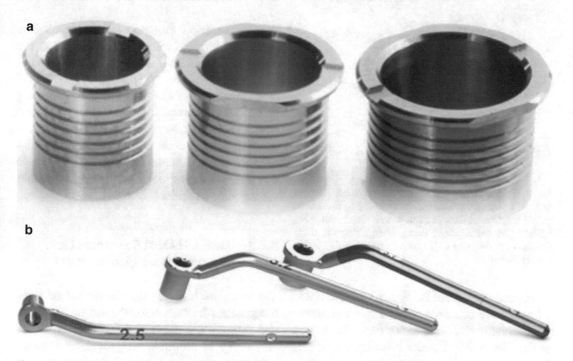

Fig. 5.15 Different sleeve diameters and their corresponding handles, from Biohorizons®

handle height and drill length selection for each implant to be placed (Fig. 5.17). Thus, some software programs offer a drilling report for printing and visualization during surgery. This can be very useful when planning multiple implant placement (Fig. 5.18).

Moreover, the addition of multiple elements increments the number of gaps. As said before, tolerance between guide and sleeve will depend on the CAM process while sleeve-handle and handle-drill tolerances will depend on implant company manufacturing and its precision [5] (Fig. 5.19).

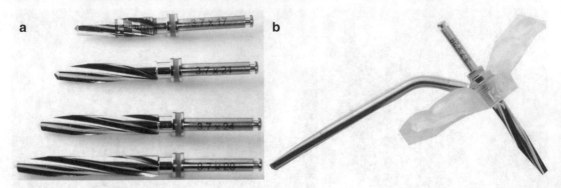

Fig. 5.16 Biohorizons® guided drilling system. Drill length variation depends on the drilling protocol indicated by the software. The length in these drills does not relate to the implant length but to an algorithm proposed by the software to achieve the desired osteotomy depth

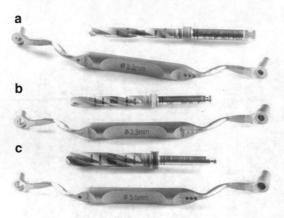

Fig. 5.17 Straumann® guided drilling system. Handles codified by color to relate to the corresponding drill. Also, handle height compensation can be visualized with either 1 colored dot (+1 mm) or 3 dots (+3 mm). Note that drills maintain their diameter along the whole active segment length

Implant placement in systems with variable offset usually demands a driver instrument that contains indication lines to determine the desired depth (Fig. 5.20). Correct visualization of this limit can be difficult in posterior regions.

To summarize, this system eases sub-crestal osteotomy preparations, offers customized offsets and avoids tissue interference during drilling. However, multiple variants have to be controlled during surgery and two hands are needed to secure both handle and drill.

5.4 Sleeveless Surgical Guides

There is a raising current of fabricating surgical templates with the sleeve incorporated into the design [6]. This idea aims to reduce gaps and thus, increase accuracy. Precision on the CAM procedure is critical to obtain a reliable drilling hole, as it has to match the instrument diameter without a metal pre-fabricated element. Surgical cassettes are the same as the ones described and used for sleeved guides. The only difference is that metal sleeve is omitted and designed within the template structure (Fig. 5.21).

5.4.1 DRILL HANDLE Systems (for Sleeveless Surgical Guides)

The template includes the sleeve that receives the handle. The system has the same advantages and pitfalls than described for sleeved guides but a gap is eliminated in order to enhance accuracy.

These templates can be printed or milled, and can be manufactured with different materials. Main reason for this is that the drill does not interact with the guide itself but with the handle. Thus, there is no risk for material derivate being driven into the osteotomy.

Implant position	Implant Art. No.	Implant	Sleeve Art. No.	Sleeve	Sleeve height	Sleeve position	Basic implant bed preparation		
							Milling cutter	Guided drill	Cylinder of drill handle
2	021.6508	BL, Ø 4.8mm RC, SLA® 8mm, Roxolid®, Loxim®	034.053V4	Ø 5.0 mm T-sleeve	5 mm	H6	Ø 4.20 mm	☰ Medium 20 mm	• +1 mm
4	021.4510	BL, Ø 4.1mm RC, SLA® 10mm, Roxolid®, Loxim®	034.053V4	Ø 5.0 mm T-sleeve	5 mm	H6	Ø 3.50 mm	☰ Long 24 mm	••• +3 mm
5	021.2512	BL, Ø 3.3mm NC, SLA® 12mm, Roxolid®, Loxim®	034.053V4	Ø 5.0 mm T-sleeve	5 mm	H6	Ø 2.80 mm	☰ Long 24 mm	• +1 mm
7	021.2512	BL, Ø 3.3mm NC, SLA® 12mm, Roxolid®, Loxim®	034.053V4	Ø 5.0 mm T-sleeve	5 mm	H6	Ø 2.80 mm	☰ Long 24 mm	• +1 mm
9	021.2512	BL, Ø 3.3mm NC, SLA® 12mm, Roxolid®, Loxim®	034.053V4	Ø 5.0 mm T-sleeve	5 mm	H6	Ø 2.80 mm	☰ Long 24 mm	• +1 mm
11	021.2512	BL, Ø 3.3mm NC, SLA® 12mm, Roxolid®, Loxim®	034.053V4	Ø 5.0 mm T-sleeve	5 mm	H6	Ø 2.80 mm	☰ Long 24 mm	• +1 mm
13	021.4510	BL, Ø 4.1mm RC, SLA® 10mm, Roxolid®, Loxim®	034.053V4	Ø 5.0 mm T-sleeve	5 mm	H6	Ø 3.50 mm	☰ Long 24 mm	••• +3 mm
15	021.6508	BL, Ø 4.8mm RC, SLA® 8mm, Roxolid®, Loxim®	034.053V4	Ø 5.0 mm T-sleeve	5 mm	H6	Ø 4.20 mm	☰ Medium 20 mm	• +1 mm

Fig. 5.18 Drilling report proposed for a multiple implant placement case. Implant and sleeve codes are indicated to place the order for the surgery. Also, offset is indicated for each implant ("Sleeve position" column; H2, H4, or H6 in this selected system), together with the length of the drill that should be used ("Guided drill" column; either Short, Medium, or Long in this system selected) and the handle compensation ("Cylinder of drill handle" column; +1 mm or +3 mm in this system selected)

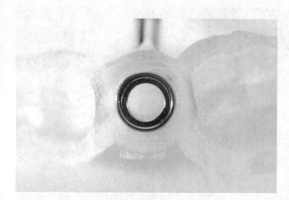

Fig. 5.19 Tolerance (gap) between sleeve and handle

Sleeve-handle tolerance reduction is also improved because friction is allowed between metal (handle) and resin (guide) material. Therefore, fit can be adjusted to reduce this gap. On the contrary, tolerance between two metal structures (metal sleeve and handle) does not allow friction and so, gap in sleeved guides has to permit friction-free fit.

5.4.2   GUIDED DRILL Systems (for Sleeveless Surgical Guides)

Drills with a guided segment are used directly into the guide, without any sleeve interposed. Tolerance is reduced to minimum and a small friction is allowed. Therefore, the use of a material which does not produce derivates is mandatory.

PMMA or PEEK materials are needed to be milled and fabricate these templates. 3D printed materials cannot be used and so, costs are increased considerably. However, a pre-fabricated

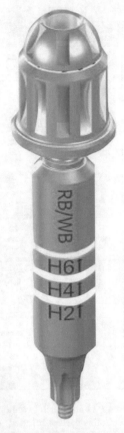

Fig. 5.20 Implant depth line indication for each sleeve offset

metal sleeve is not needed and cost can be reduced in this aspect (Fig. 5.22).

Moreover, these guides can be designed to fit multiple holes in reduced spaces, where sleeve placement is not possible. Also, hole design can adapt to tissue architecture, unlike with pre-fabricated sleeves. Although not a frequent problem with regular sleeved guides, there is no risk of sleeve detachment while drilling with these templates.

These guides tend to be more rigid and less flexible because of the material used to fabricate them. So, template bending is minimized. Additionally, tissue interference can always be a problem whenever using guided drills, with or without sleeves.

5.5 Pilot Drill Surgical Guides

Some implant companies offer a small diameter sleeve destined to the first drill, usually known as pilot drill. The sleeve inner diameter wanders around 2 or 2.2 mm. Its use is limited to narrow spaces, where a regular diameter sleeve cannot fit. Also, they are used for osteotomy depth and direction pre-preparations, before continuing with a tra-

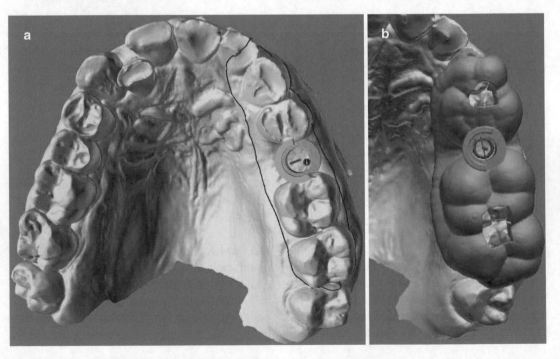

Fig. 5.21 Sleeve is included into template design

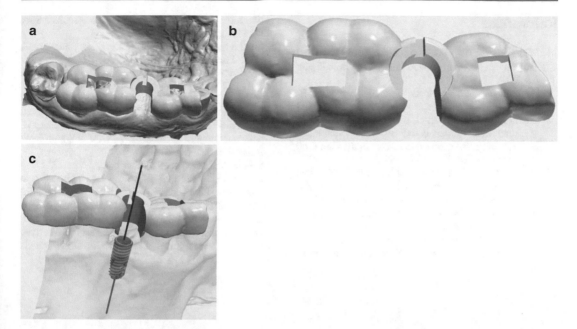

Fig. 5.22 Sleeveless guide design for Osstem® guided drill system. This system provides an open window in the buccal aspect to facilitate drill positioning, especially in a posterior area, and improve irrigation. Caution must be taken to avoid weak palatal/lingual areas within this design

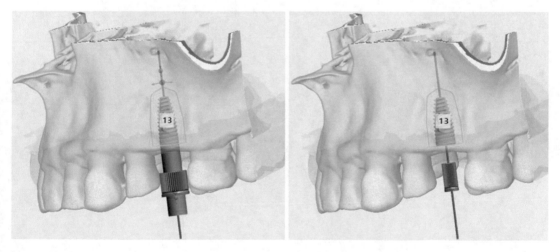

Fig. 5.23 Virtual implant planning for a fully guided (left) or a pilot drilling protocol (right), in which the sleeve contains only information for the initial (pilot) drill

ditional free-handed surgical protocol (Fig. 5.23). Moreover, these templates are often used to mark implant position in simultaneous bone regenerative surgery, where final implant bed preparation demands direct vision and free-hand control in order to preserve existing bone [7].

Implants cannot be driven with these templates; only pilot drill can be used. Nevertheless, these guides can help rapid implant distribution in extended edentulous sites, in cases where the surgeon prefers conventional free-hand protocol [8].

As pilot drill templates use a metal sleeve, manufacturing can be accomplished either with 3D printers or milling machines. All template materials are suitable.

References

1. Widmann G, Bale RJ. Accuracy in computer-aided implant surgery: a review. Int J Oral Maxillofac Implants. 2006;21(2):305–13.
2. Derksen W, Wismeijer D, Flügge T, Hassan B, Tahmaseb A. The accuracy of computer-guided implant surgery with tooth-supported, digitally designed drill guides based on CBCT and intra-oral scanning. A prospective cohort study. Clin Oral Implants Res. 2019;30(10):1005–15.
3. Lee DH, An SY, Hong MH, Jeon KB, Lee KB. Accuracy of a direct drill-guiding system with minimal tolerance of surgical instruments used for implant surgery: a prospective clinical study. J Adv Prosthodont. 2016;8(3):207–13.
4. Naziri E, Schramm A, Wilde F. Accuracy of computer-assisted implant placement with insertion templates. GMS Interdiscip Plast Reconstr Surg DGPW. 2016;5:Doc15.
5. Sigcho López DA, García I, Da Silva Salomao G, Cruz Laganá D. Potential deviation factors affecting stereolithographic surgical guides. Implant Dent. 2019;28(1):68–73.
6. Tallarico M, Kim Y-J, Cocchi F, Martinolli M, Meloni SM. Accuracy of newly developed sleeve-designed templates for insertion of dental implants: a prospective multicenters clinical trial. Clin Implant Dent Relat Res. 2019;21:108–13.
7. Schulz MC, Hofmann F, Range U, Lauer G, Haim D. Pilot-drill guided vs. full-guided implant insertion in artificial mandibles-a prospective laboratory study in fifth-year dental students. Int J Implant Dent. 2019;5(1):23.
8. Behneke A, Burwinkel M, Behneke N. Factors influencing transfer accuracy of cone beam CT-derived template-based implant placement. Clin Oral Implants Res. 2011;23(4):416–23.

Implant Placement, Accuracy Assessment and Literature Review

6

Diego A. Coccorullo and Nicolás A. Rubio

6.1 Introduction

This chapter explains implant driving options and assesses its accuracy related, followed by an attempt to include a literature review regarding considerations for improving accuracy in implant guided surgery.

Similar to template design, the implant placement method selected is also related with outcome accuracy. Moreover, other considerations can be taken into account for obtaining more or less predictable results.

Among surgical guided protocols, different options are available for implant placement. On one hand, virtual planning can be transferred to the clinical situation by guiding osteotomies and allowing implant to be placed free-handed. On the other hand, a fully guided protocol can be achieved by guiding both osteotomy and implant insertion through the guide. Additionally, another option has been described previously (see Sect. 5.5, Chap. 5), in which only the first drill is guided by the template. Decision on what protocol should be used will depend on clinical situation, surgeon experience and preferences.

As assumed, overall accuracy assessment is stablished by the possibility of transferring virtual implant position to the jaws. Therefore, whenever free-handed steps are included in the protocol, more deviation from the initial plan can be expected. This variation is measured by analyzing angular deviation (in degrees) and linear deviations, in the apex and in the coronal aspect of the implant (in mm). Implant height discrepancy can be also considered among literature.

In an attempt to justify the use of virtual planning, some authors have tried to compare guided techniques with conventional implant placement. Although results are satisfactory, comparison tends to be difficult, as non-guided surgery does not have a pre-planned implant position to compare with. To solve this issue, virtual implant planning is also performed in these cases in order to help clinicians visualize the desired future implant position. Nevertheless, results cannot be objectively measured.

It is important to highlight that implant survival rates tend to be 95–100% when using static Computer Aided Implant Surgery (sCAIS). This information proves that these protocols can be validated as a confident procedure in terms of osseointegration.

6.2 Implant Driving Options

Guided implant surgery is scientific and clinically validated for daily practice and has shown implant survival rates comparable to conventional

D. A. Coccorullo (✉) · N. A. Rubio
Universidad de Buenos Aires,
Ciudad Autónoma de Buenos Aires, Argentina

© Springer Nature Switzerland AG 2021
J. M. Galante, N. A. Rubio (eds.), *Digital Dental Implantology*,
https://doi.org/10.1007/978-3-030-65947-9_6

procedures [1]. However, it requires training and expertise to reach highly predictable results.

Static computer aided implant surgery (sCAIS) gives surgeons the chance to perform previous planning and accurately transfer it to the patient afterwards. Following strict indications, clinician should arrive to the planned situation. Although sCAIS seems a straightforward protocol, expertise is necessary to assess every clinical situation. Among most common clinical decisions, implant driving tends to be the most variable option during surgery.

Therefore, three basic options are presented for the clinician to select: pilot drilling, guided and fully guided protocols.

6.2.1 Pilot Drilling Protocol

Perhaps the simplest guided protocol is pilot drilling, a technique that involves designing a template to guide only the first drill, usually known as pilot drill. This instrument has a diameter that often ranges from 1.8 to 2.2 mm. Following this initial osteotomy, template is discarded and drilling protocol is finished conventionally.

There are two ways of performing this protocol. One is designing a conventional sleeved template and limiting the osteotomy to the first drill. This can be useful for those implant systems that

do not offer a pilot drilling kit. Another option is designing the osteotomy protocol specifically for a narrower "pilot" sleeve (available in some implant systems). This can be useful in narrow edentulous spaces (Fig. 6.1).

Major applications of this procedure are: sleeve diameter reduction for narrow edentulous spaces, simplifying surgical kits (Fig. 6.2), improving manual control over osteotomies when necessary (i.e.: grafted sites), rapid determining implant distribution and angulation in extended edentulous spaces and stablishing initial implant preparation in ridges prior to simultaneous grafting techniques.

To clarify, this protocol will work as it has been described as long as further drilling is required; that is, if more than one drill is needed for implant bed preparation. On the contrary, the use of very narrow implants, or mini-implants, requiring only one drill should be considered as a guided protocol.

6.2.2 Free-Handed Implant Placement (Guided Protocol)

Taking a step ahead into guided surgery, osteotomies can be performed in a sequential way until reaching the moment of implant placement. Contrary to the previous protocol, drilling is completed through the template but implant is driven manually.

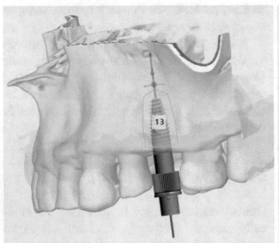 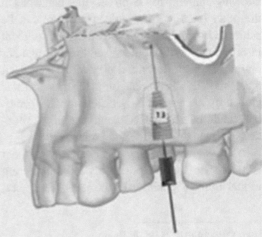

Fig. 6.1 Implant planned for a guided protocol (left) and for a pilot drilling protocol (right). Both planning can be used for pilot drilling sequence only

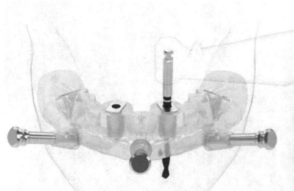
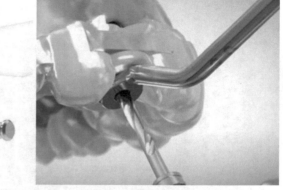

Fig. 6.2 Nobel® pilot drill surgical kit option (left), suitable for narrow spaces and for reducing instrument costs. BioHorizons® full guided surgical kit used to perform a pilot drilling protocol (right), using the same template design that is used for fully guided protocols

As manual osteotomy is not allowed here, the surgeon must be confident about guided drilling; that is, previous assessment should take place to verify that what has been planned is perfectly related to the clinical scenario. Whenever this situation does not meet previous planning, guided drilling protocol should be aborted to proceed manually.

Main indication of this protocol is the need for controlling implant driving maneuver. Parameters as implant inclination, tooth proximity and depth position can be therefore assessed by the clinician without template interference. Moreover, as described in Chap. 5, sub-crestal implant position can impede wider instruments from reaching the desired depth. In those cases, implant can be either driven manually or partially guided with manual final adjustment.

6.2.3   Fully Guided Protocol

If during virtual planning, the process has been smooth and straightforward; and if during surgery, template has perfectly fitted and clinical situation meets what has been planned, fully guided protocol is clearly the best indication. Is with the use of this technique that sCAIS exhibits its major benefits (Fig. 6.3).

Implant insertion is done with template assistance. To achieve this, two different instruments can be used. Some implant systems offer "guided" implants with a special mounter attached to them, suitable for this protocol. Said implants had to be ordered specifically and had to be selected within the software as well. Clinician must be aware that both variables of implant mounter (guided and conventional) can sometimes be found in the same virtual library. Mistakes made on implant mounter selection within the software can deliver improper vertical final position of the implant. Main disadvantage of this option is the need of stock duplication in the office.

Other implant systems provide an adapted driver tool for guided surgery, different from the conventional one, that engages the implant mounter (or even the implant itself). This instrument has a guided portion that relates to the sleeve, helping clinicians use the same implant than used for manual procedures (Fig. 6.4).

Some brands justify the incorporation of said special guided mounter to their implants by stating that it improves accuracy. While this can be inferred, due to the stiffness of the implant/mounter connection and the guided portion being offered by this same mounter, some authors have failed to find relevant differences in terms of accuracy, when comparing it to guided adapter drivers [2].

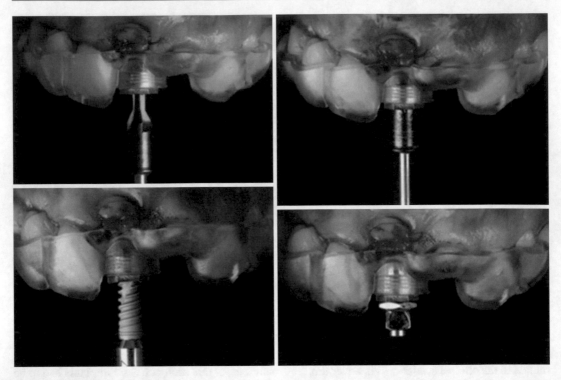

Fig. 6.3 Clinical case using a fully guided protocol

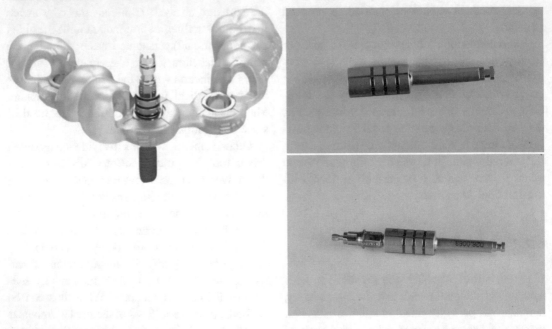

Fig. 6.4 Guided implant with incorporated special mounter (left) and guided adapter for conventional implant mounters (right) from Straumann®

6.2.4 Accuracy Assessment

Younes et al. [3] evaluated final implant position in a randomized clinical trial (RCT), comparing conventional implant surgery with pilot drilling and fully guided protocols. Assessment included implant angular deviation (AnD), error at entry point (EP), and apex deviation (ApD) (Fig. 6.5).

Additionally, Behneke et al. [4] also assessed the same variables in another RCT, but included a free-handed implant placement test group (guided protocol) and avoided a conventional implant surgery control group. Both studies results can be seen in Tables 6.1 and 6.2.

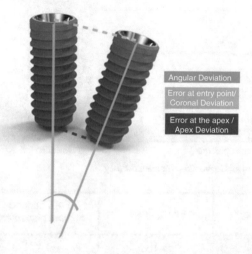

Fig. 6.5   Implant position assessment design

Outcomes indicate that, as guided sequence is followed, accuracy is improved. So, fully guided protocol appears to be the most reliable technique, followed by free-handed placement and pilot drilling (Table 6.1). It is important to outline that all virtual guided procedures threw considerable better results than conventional implant surgery (Table 6.2). Moreover, one study [3] incorporated an interesting secondary result regarding final prosthetic outcome. Although all crowns in the study were planned to be screw-retained, cemented restorations had to be delivered in the following cases:

- 5 of 26 (19.2%) of conventional implant surgery cases.
- 1 of 24 (4.2%) of pilot guide cases.
- 0 of 21 (0%) of fully guided cases.

Differences can be found between these two similar studies. Although Behneke et al. study [4] was performed in 2011, it throws better results

Table 6.1   Accuracy outcomes of the three variants of the guided protocols, extracted from Behneke et al. [4]

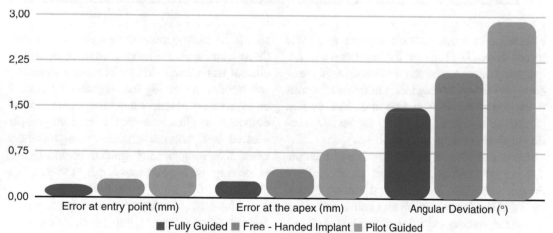

	Fully guided	Free-handed implant placement	Pilot guided
Error at entry point (mm)	0.21	0.30	0.52
Error at the apex (mm)	0.28	0.47	0.81
Angular Deviation (°)	1.49	2.06	2.91

Table 6.2 Accuracy outcomes comparing guided protocols with conventional implant surgery, extracted from Younes et al. [3]

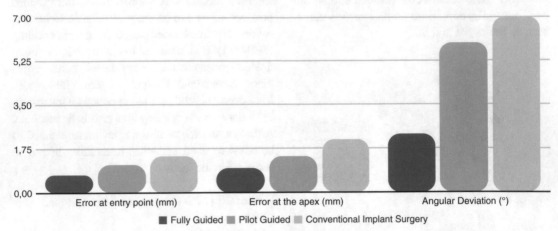

	Fully guided	Pilot guided	Free-handed implant placement
Error at entry point (mm)	0.73	1.12	1.45
Error at the apex (mm)	0.97	1.43	2.11
Angular Deviation (°)	2.30	5.95	6.99

in terms of accuracy when compared to a more recent study [3]. However, the latest uses a protocol comparable to the one described in this textbook and shows homogeneity in terms of results when compared to Tahmaseb et al. last revision [5]. Mean outcomes shown by the review mentioned above can be seen in Table 6.3.

Values of EP and ApD below 2 mm are considered acceptable for clinical practice. Even though variations can be found among studies included in this revision, worst clinical outcomes, measured at the apex of the implants, were 2 mm for fully guided cases and 5 mm for conventional implant surgery [3]. Thus, prosthetic and biological risks can be minimized with sCAIS.

Bover-Ramos et al. [6] also compared partially (free-handed) and fully guided protocols in clinical, cadaver, and in vitro studies. Among their conclusions, they found that in vitro studies

tend to be more optimistic than the rest, as they throw more accurate results when compared to clinical and cadaver studies. Thus, this statement can serve as a warning for surgeons to consider an extra safety margin when transposing in vitro outcomes to clinical reality. Above all, results showed a significantly accuracy improvement when following a fully guided protocol, that is, driving the implant assisted by the template (Tables 6.4, 6.5, 6.6, 6.7, and 6.8.

Technology development and professional understanding of the digital workflow certainly generate accuracy improvement and treatment predictability. Therefore, most recent clinical studies (from Behneke et al. [4] to date) [3, 7–10] show values ranging from: 1.4 to 5.95° for AnD; 0.43 to 1.12 mm for EP; and 0.67 to 1.43 for ApD. These outcomes are all extrapolated from partially edentulous cases.

Table 6.3 Tahmaseb et al. [5] revision main outcomes regarding implant final position using guided protocols, both in partially and fully edentulous patients

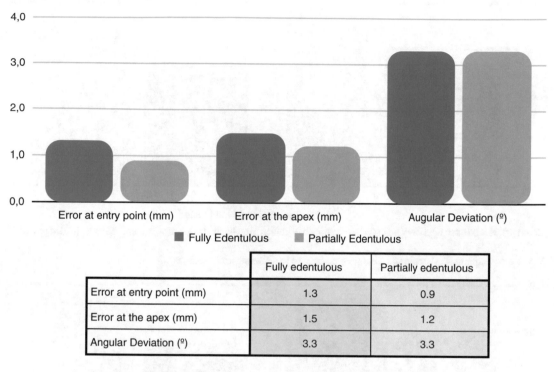

	Fully edentulous	Partially edentulous
Error at entry point (mm)	1.3	0.9
Error at the apex (mm)	1.5	1.2
Angular Deviation (º)	3.3	3.3

Table 6.4 Comparison between different study types

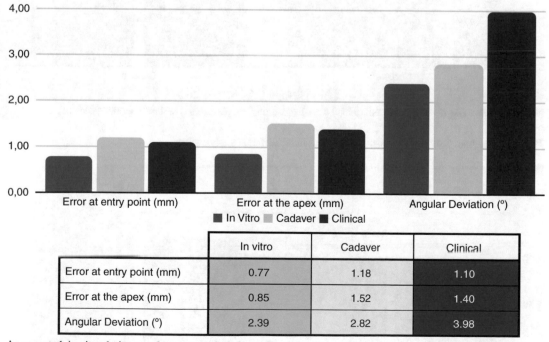

	In vitro	Cadaver	Clinical
Error at entry point (mm)	0.77	1.18	1.10
Error at the apex (mm)	0.85	1.52	1.40
Angular Deviation (°)	2.39	2.82	3.98

As expected, in vitro designs tend to more optimistic results

Table 6.5 Implant final position assessment associated to different study designs

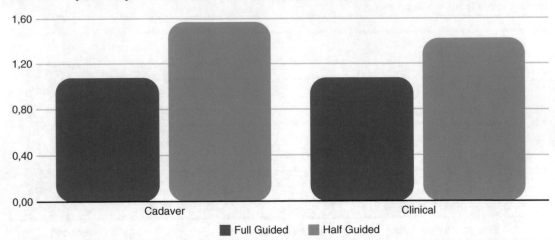

Coronal deviation or error at entry point (EP) comparing half guided (free-handed implant placement) and fully guided protocols

Table 6.6 Implant final position assessment associated to different study designs

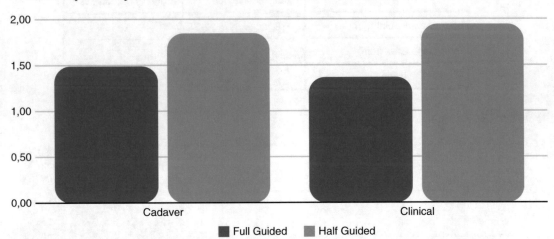

Apical deviation (ApD) comparing half guided (free-handed implant placement) and fully guided protocols

Table 6.7 Implant final position assessment associated to different study designs

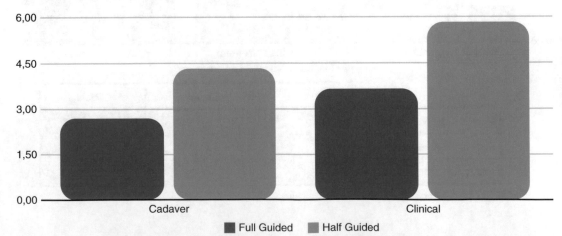

Angular deviation (AnD) comparing half guided (free-handed implant placement) and fully guided protocols

Table 6.8 Implant final position assessment associated to different study designs

		Full guided	Half guided
Error at entry point (mm)	Cadaver	1.07	1.56
	Clinical	1.08	1.42
Error at the apex (mm)	Cadaver	1.47	1.84
	Clinical	1.35	1.92
Angular deviation (°)	Cadaver	2.69	4.30
	Clinical	3.62	5.82

6.3 Considerations for Achieving Accuracy During Virtual Planning

6.3.1 Considerations for CAI Procedures

When considering CAI procedures, image acquisition involves surface scans and tomography images.

First of all, when wax-up type is analyzed, no differences are found between analog and virtual wax-up (direct or indirect wax-up) [11]; so, both techniques are suitable.

Second, small differences are found in surface topography and volumetric analysis when comparing different intraoral and extraoral scanners. For the acquisition of STL files, Renne et al. [12] analyzed two aspects of accuracy: precision (repeatable and consistent scanning) and trueness (correct dimensions of the scanned object). In relation to these two variants, EOs had the best performance in almost all groups analyzed. Also, in their study, they came to the conclusion that IOs had different performance according to the scanning method, (sextant or a full arch), and this had direct relation with the time needed by each device. Thus, although trueness and precision were widely evaluated, many factors affect clinical performance of IOs and therefore, deeper investigation is needed. Each IOs system presents advantages for some clinical situation while some are more suitable for other purposes. Focus should be made on the influence of implant accuracy depending on the scanning method, but this is difficult to assess, as many variables need to be taken into account.

Flugge et al. [13] found more accuracy in intraoral scanning samples when compared to extraoral scanning, both using IOs and EOs for model scanning (in vitro). Kiatkroekkrai et al. [9] reported minimum differences in implant final position when using surface scans obtained either with IOS or EOS. IOS scans were more prone to achieve more accurate results, but this difference was not significant. Other authors failed to find differences related to the scanner used [11] or found a tendency towards finding a smaller deviation when intraoral scanner was used; although not significant [8].

To continue with CBCT imaging acquisition, according to Patterson et al. [14], patient movement during CBCT scanning can significantly influence implant apical and coronal final position. Thus, consistent protocols must be used to enhance CBCT imaging in the search for precision within the digital planning. Nevertheless, the study by Patterson et al. [14] used a 70 seconds parameter to complete the CBCT scan, while nowadays this study can be performed in a shorter period of time. Special considerations should be taken by the clinician whenever prescribing CBCT examinations to elderly patients or patients with difficulties to remain still over a considerable period of time. Moreover, distortions in implant final position found in this article can be explained by the use of a final tomography to measure results. More recent studies proclaim the use of intraoral scanning to obtain these results, rather than CBCT images.

Flugge et al. [15] also evaluated how segmentation influences final image obtained from CBCT. For that means, they compared manual and automatic segmentation for the production of a 3D render. Four examiners found considerable better results towards the manual procedure, as it improved surface definition and sharpness, facilitating image merging process. However, one of the examiners showed poor results for both procedures that can potentially alter significance of said outcomes. Nevertheless, manual segmentation can be recommended if wanting to get the most out of the CBCT rendering (Fig. 6.6).

Furthermore, this latest study [15] also analyzed the influence of the amount of metallic res-

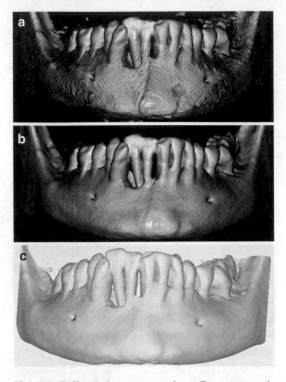

Fig. 6.6 Different jaw segmentations. From automatic rendering (**a**) to parameter adjustments (**b**) and manual segmentation (**c**). 3D reconstruction quality can influence the merging process

torations present in the jaw for obtaining a neat digital image with CBCT scanning. Artifact produced by jaws containing more than six metallic restorations showed more deviations when merging images. Thus, this is a factor to be considered when indicating a virtual planning procedure (Fig. 6.7). This statement is in concordance with Derksen et al. recommendations [7], who also found significant improvement in the merging process whenever 7 or more un-restored teeth were available to do the matching.

6.3.2 Considerations for CAD Procedures

Incorrect template design can alter final implant position. So, some considerations have to be outlined. First of all, as recommended in Chap. 4, guides presenting distal extensions should be reinforced by the means of lateral bars (Fig. 6.8) or material thickening. Derksen et al. in vivo [7] and El Kholy et al. in vitro [16] found a negative relation between template cantilever and implant accurate position. However, when considering a

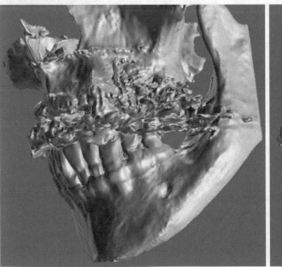
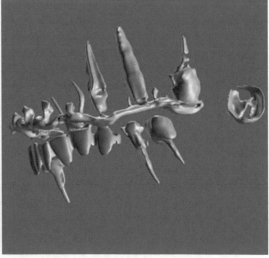

Fig. 6.7 Increased presence of metallic restorations produces scattering and compromises image visualization (left). Although artifact can be diminished, metallic objects remain visible despite tissue density adjustments (right)

3-unit bridge, distal implant placement was less precise than the mesial one. Therefore, in that cases, initial mesial implant placement can be a suitable option for diminishing template deformation during distal implant osteotomy.

Other interesting aspect was also described by Derksen et al. [7] when assessing the influence of teeth crowding in implant accuracy. Although fitting of the template was always more arduous in these cases, no discrepancies were found in relation to final implant position when compared to templates fit on aligned dentition.

El Kholy et al. [16] also verified differences in implant final position when comparing implants placed between teeth (tooth-supported templates) and implants placed in distal extensions (combined templates). This difference increased as the implant position was more distal, i.e., tooth 26 less precise than tooth 25. Moreover, this outcome was not significantly registered for the

angular deviation variable. The authors relate this finding to the lack of support that generates template tilting and bending.

On the other hand, El Kholy et al. [16] assessed implant precision in relation to the extent of guide support and retention, in tooth-supported templates and single implant cases (in vitro). Accuracy was improved whenever three teeth were used to support the guide in the posterior area. In comparison, at least four teeth were needed to increase accuracy in the anterior zone (Fig. 6.9). Although reducing the extension of the guide can reduce costs and facilitate manufacturing, minimum extension has to ensure proper stability.

El Kholy et al. [2] found differences between implant final position and its macro-design. Conical shaped implants obtained better results than parallel wall ones. Authors associated this phenomenon to the difference between surgical instruments (drill design).

Furthermore, as mentioned before, no significant difference was found between implants driven with a specific guided mounter or with regular mounters and an adapted driver [2]. Thus, no justification on the use on guided implants can be made.

6.3.3   Considerations for CAM Procedures

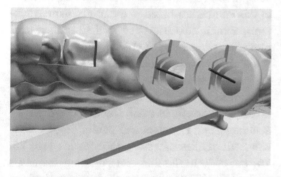

Fig. 6.8 Lateral bar reinforcement for distal extensions helps minimize template bending during osteotomies

Many tips for 3D printing procedures have been analyzed in Chap. 3. Despite being a critical step,

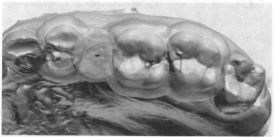 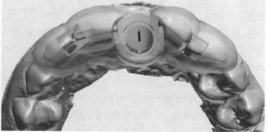

Fig. 6.9 Minimum template extension recommended for accuracy improvement involves including three posterior (left) or four anterior teeth (right)

not many articles relate manufacturing procedures with final clinical outcomes.

Both DLP and SLA printers showed great performances when assessing drill fitting in sleeve-free guides and comparing them to multi-jet systems [17]. Additionally, no differences were found between DLP and SLA printer outcomes for this variable. However, Oh et al. [17] also demonstrated deficient mucosal adaptation when comparing DLP and SLA printers with poly-jet systems, for distal extended templates.

Also, Herschdorfer et al. [18] studied final implant position, in vitro, using different printed templates. They did not find significant differences in any measured variable between a multi-jet printer (ProJet 3500 by 3DSystems®), a poly-jet printer (Object Eden 260vs by Stratasys®) and a stereolithographic method (Form 2 by FormLabs®). Although outcomes were more precise and accurate for the multi-jet printer, all three methods succeeded in delivering acceptable clinical results.

Additionally, Henprasert et al. [19] measured in vitro precision of implants placed in the same position with templates fabricated either with subtractive or additive methods. No significant differences were found in none of the eight variables measured.

6.4 Considerations for Achieving Accuracy During Clinical Procedures

6.4.1 Template Accuracy

Taking into account last literature reviews [5, 6, 20], clinical behavior of all templates has successfully reported excellent outcomes regarding reproducibility of virtual implant planning. Even though some authors [5, 6, 20] do not specify what type of template is more precise, when analyzed together, overall performance fits into acceptable clinical margins of 2 mm deviation. Biggest errors have been reported for edentulous maxilla cases by Verhamme et al. [21–23], from 4 and up to 8 mm.

Many variables can influence outcome; thus, individual details need to be addressed in every single step of the planning and execution. As angular deviations are the less significant aspects among the variables assessed through literature, errors such as apical and coronal linear deviations can be adjudicated to image superimposing procedures when assessing results, rather than adjudicated to template design.

6.4.2 Drilling System Accuracy

Most investigation regarding drilling accuracy is done in vitro, by testing instrument movement and capturing it with optical instruments (Fig. 6.10). Using this method, longer drills are normally related to greater pantographic deviations [24]. However, Derksen et al. [7] found more precise results in implants of 12 mm length, compared to shorter ones. A possible explanation to this can be attributed to the use of handle systems, which also has been said to reduce drill movement compared to guided drill systems as it is stabilized by the operator second hand.

Regardless what implant length is needed and the drilling system it uses, there are two variables than sometimes can be modified to enhance accuracy; that is: offset and guiding tube extension. All studies assessing instruments [10, 25, 26] coincide in the fact that precision increases as the offset (distance from the implant platform to the sleeve) is reduced. So, as a general rule, offset should always be as minimum as possible. Moreover, as the guiding tube (portion of the template/handle system that is guiding the drill) is longer, the osteotomy becomes more precise and lateral movement is reduced [25]. So, increasing the guiding tube can be achieved either by selecting a higher sleeve or a higher compensating handle.

Fang et al. [10] recommended the use of an extra-long key handle for the pilot drill, which is, according to them, the most critical step in the osteotomy (Fig. 6.11). This option can be suit-

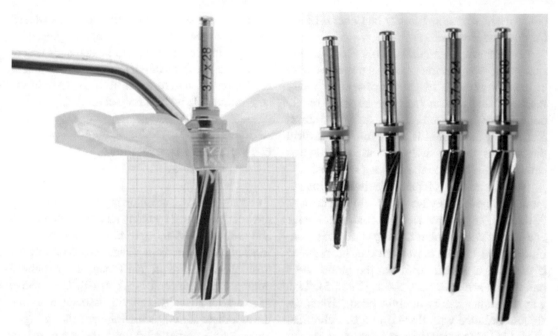

Fig. 6.10 Instrument lateral movement experiment, registered in a millimeter paper (left). Increasing drill length provokes more lateral displacement

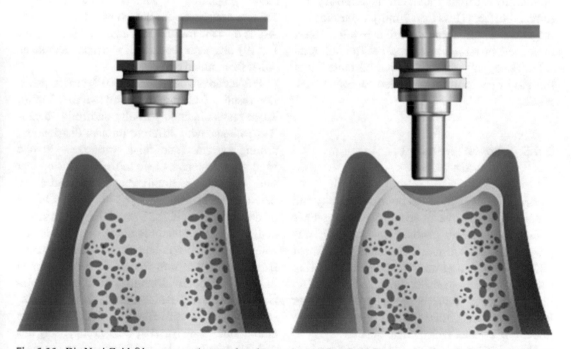

Fig. 6.11 Dio Navi Guide® key system. An extra-long key can be used for pilot drilling, as described in Fang's protocol [10]

able for anterior sites but may be rather difficult for the posterior area.

In summary, longer drills, shorter handles and shorter sleeves generate more lateral movement of the instrument. Also, higher offsets indirectly increase drill length and so, increase pantographic deviation of the instrument. One study [26] stated that lateral movement is also promoted as drill diameter is progressively increased. This was equally tested for different implant systems.

Additionally, tolerance between instruments is another key factor affecting accuracy. Although not many studies compare sleeve and sleeveless templates, Koop et al. [25], concluded that lateral movement can be reduced if the sleeve is printed within the guide and a handle is used (see Sect. 5.4.1, Chap. 5). That way, tolerance can be diminished significantly. In concordance with these findings, Schneider et al. [26] also revealed that tolerances greater than 0.1 mm between sleeve and drill had significant influence on instrument deviation in offsets higher than 7 mm. On the contrary, for reduced offsets (less than 7 mm), tolerances of 0.1 and 0.2 mm showed similar results. Here, the offset variable played another fundamental role. Thus, to conclude, it can be stated that the sum of variables is needed to control the result.

6.4.3 Patient Anatomy Considerations

Derksen et al. [7] measured bone topography and density roles in overall accuracy. Among their findings, whenever cortical interference was present, angular deviation was increased. About 40% more deviation was found when comparing cortical bone to medullar tissue. However, no differences were found between upper and lower jaw as inaccuracy only seemed to be related to implant in contact with cortical bone.

In concordance, several studies failed to prove differences between arches [4, 10, 14].

Moreover, no differences in implant final position were found between native and regenerated bone [7], but significant difference was indeed found between immediate implants placed in freshly extracted sockets and healed sites (about 50% more linear deviation and 100% more angular deviation), based on an in vitro study in the anterior maxilla by El Kholy et al. [16].

6.5 Literature Review Conclusions

Accuracy assessment following implant planning has been addressed by many authors, both in vitro and clinically. Although almost all of them showed positive outcomes regarding final implant position, a paradigm shift can be visualized among studies since 2014 [3, 7–10]. This change of work philosophy can be associated to the development of new technology and the strengthening of the digital workflow; the same as proposed in this textbook: CAI—CAD—CAM. This new concept also stablishes study designs that are more compatible to what is done nowadays. Thus, more recent studies show more accurate results than the former ones analyzed [2, 7, 8, 10, 17, 19] and also tend to use printed templates rather than milled ones.

Publications made since 2010 report precision results of 1.5 mm or less (down to 0.2 mm). These results include partially and fully edentulous patients, with different implant distribution, drilling systems, and other variables. On one hand, these outcomes lead to the conclusion that said protocols are highly predictable and allow the surgeon to achieve great accuracy. On the other hand, according to overall findings, a safety margin of 1.5 mm should always be considered when implant placement is planned virtually. Additionally, a 2 mm margin is recommended for avoiding noble structures, such as the inferior dental nerve. Bover-Ramos et al. [6] outlined the lack of vertical apical deviation results among studies analyzed by their group, being this variable important to stablish this margin with confidence.

Taking into account these parameters, every clinician should evaluate the possibility for flapless surgery by assessing bone availability, safety margins, and soft tissue considerations. sCAIS is not equivalent to flapless surgery and this statement should be highlighted.

Finally, angular deviations found within the literature round about 3.3° for implant final position, validating the use of this technology for predictable prosthetic outcomes. Nevertheless, multiple implant placement accumulates multiple angular deviations and so, immediate restoration cannot always find a proper fit. At the present time, virtual implant planning and simultaneous prosthetic restoration needs to rely on implant final position rather than virtual implant position.

6.5.1 Accuracy Related Tips

Some tips collected from literature review are presented here. Most clinical tips had already been addressed through chapter development.

- According to Derksen et al. in vivo [7] and El Kholy et al. in vitro [16], distal extensions are sites that deliver the worst results regarding precision. Thus, initial mesial implant placement can help stabilize the template for distal osteotomy preparations, as said inaccuracy is attributed to the increment of the template cantilever and consequent bending (Fig. 6.12).
- As briefly mentioned in Chap. 4, whenever having a muco-supported (or combined) template, anesthesia should not be performed

extensively in all sites to be treated, as this can alter template seating by causing tissue swelling [5] (Fig. 6.12).

- Also, regarding soft tissue support, Schnutenhaus et al. [27] specified that if tissue thickness is greater than 3.5 mm, a flap needs to be raised to reduce the influence of flap thickness on accuracy.

6.5.2 New Tendencies for Accuracy Assessment

In one of the latest revisions, Tahmaseb et al. [5] selected studies ranging from 2008 to 2016. Analyzing their selection, it can be seen that the majority of the study designs used post-operative CBCT to assess final implant position (19 from 20 publications selected). As it can be assumed, 3D reconstruction provided by CBCT and implant artifact can jeopardize correct image merging between implant planning and implant final position (Fig. 6.13). Moreover, recent vertiginous growth of digital technology regarding scanners and their wide-spread usage eases this problem. Final implant position can nowadays be assessed by surface scan and the use of scan bodies. Therefore, more recent studies are based on surface scan comparison and are, naturally, delivering better results. Although this study design helps improve accuracy and avoids the need for unnecessary radiation exposure, new measurements meet previous outcomes, validating the whole process.

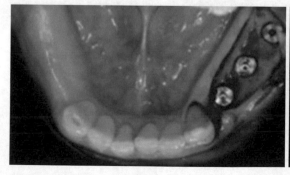
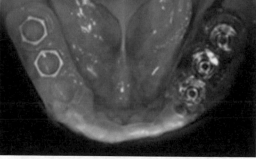

Fig. 6.12 Anesthesia is not perfused in the right quadrant to avoid tissue swelling and enhance guide adaptation (left). After implant placement, implant mounts help contralateral guide stability (right). Mesial implant should be first positioned to secure the guide for the following distal ones

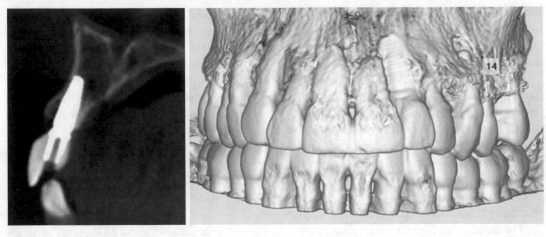

Fig. 6.13 Implant final position assessment using CBCT images. At least minimum artifact can be expected from the implant image (left). Also, 3D rendering (right) can vary as described previously in this chapter

As a reference, it can be mentioned that Nickenig [24] suggested the use of a sophisticated coordinate method to measure results and so, avoid patient over exposure to radiographic radiation. This method can be easily replaced nowadays by intraoral scanners.

References

1. Tahmaseb A, Wismeijer D, Coucke W, Derksen W. Computer technology applications in surgical implant dentistry: a systematic review. Int J Oral Maxillofac Implants. 2014;29(Suppl):25–42.
2. El Kholy K, Ebenezer S, Wittneben JG, Lazarin R, Rousson D, Buser D. Influence of implant macrodesign and insertion connection technology on the accuracy of static computer-assisted implant surgery. Clin Implant Dent Relat Res. 2019;21(5):1073–9.
3. Younes F, Cosyn J, De Bruyckere T, Cleymaet R, Bouckaert E, Eghbali A. A randomized controlled study on the accuracy of free-handed, pilot-drill guided and fully guided implant surgery in partially edentulous patients. J Clin Periodontol. 2018;45(6):721–32.
4. Behneke A, Burwinkel M, Behneke N. Factors influencing transfer accuracy of cone beam CT-derived template-based implant placement. Clin Oral Implants Res. 2012;23(4):416–23.
5. Tahmaseb A, Wu V, Wismeijer D, Coucke W, Evans C. The accuracy of static computer-aided implant surgery: a systematic review and meta-analysis. Clin Oral Implants Res. 2018;29:416.
6. Bover-Ramos F, Viña-Almunia J, Cervera-Ballester J, Peñarrocha-Diago M, García-Mira B. Accuracy of implant placement with computer-guided surgery: a systematic review and meta-analysis compar-

ing cadaver, clinical, and in vitro studies. Int J Oral Maxillofac Implants. 2018;33(1):101–15.
7. Derksen W, Wismeijer D, Flügge T, Hassan B, Tahmaseb A. The accuracy of computer-guided implant surgery with tooth-supported, digitally designed drill guides based on CBCT and intraoral scanning. A prospective cohort study. Clin Oral Implants Res. 2019;30(10):1005–15.
8. Schneider D, Sancho-Puchades M, Mir-Marí J, Mühlemann S, Jung R, Hämmerle CA. Randomized controlled clinical trial comparing conventional and computer-assisted implant planning and placement in partially edentulous patients. Part 4: accuracy of implant placement. Int J Periodontics Restorative Dent. 2019;39(4):e111–22.
9. Kiatkroekkrai P, Takolpuckdee C, Subbalekha K, Mattheos N, Pimkhaokham A. Accuracy of implant position when placed using static computer-assisted implant surgical guides manufactured with two different optical scanning techniques: a randomized clinical trial. Int J Oral Maxillofac Surg. 2020;49(3):377–83.
10. Fang Y, An X, Jeong SM, Choi BH. Accuracy of computer-guided implant placement in anterior regions. J Prosthet Dent. 2019;121(5):836–42.
11. Tallarico M, Xhanari E, Kim YJ, Cocchi F, Martinolli M, Alushi A, Baldoni EE, Meloni SM. Accuracy of computer-assisted template-based implant placement using conventional impression and scan model or intraoral digital impression: a randomised controlled trial with 1 year of follow-up. Int J Oral Implantol (Berl). 2019;12(2):197–206.
12. Renne W, Ludlow M, Fryml J, Schurch Z, Mennito A, Kessler R, Lauer A. Evaluation of the accuracy of 7 digital scanners: an in vitro analysis based on 3-dimensional comparisons. J Prosthet Dent. 2017;118(1):36–42.
13. Flügge TV, Schlager S, Nelson K, Nahles S, Metzger MC. Precision of intraoral digital dental impressions

with iTero and extraoral digitization with the iTero and a model scanner. Am J Orthod Dentofac Orthop. 2013;144(3):471–8.

14. Pettersson A, Komiyama A, Hultin M, Näsström K, Klinge B. Accuracy of virtually planned and template guided implant surgery on edentate patients. Clin Implant Dent Relat Res. 2012;14(4):527–37.

15. Flügge T, Derksen W, Te Poel J, Hassan B, Nelson K, Wismeijer D. Registration of cone beam computed tomography data and intraoral surface scans – a prerequisite for guided implant surgery with CAD/CAM drilling guides. Clin Oral Implants Res. 2017;28(9):1113–8.

16. El Kholy K, Lazarin R, Janner SFM, Faerber K, Buser R, Buser D. Influence of surgical guide support and implant site location on accuracy of static computer-assisted implant surgery. Clin Oral Implants Res. 2019;30(11):1067–75.

17. Oh KC, Park JM, Shim JS, Kim JH, Kim JE, Kim JH. Assessment of metal sleeve-free 3D-printed implant surgical guides. Dent Mater. 2019;35(3):468–76.

18. Herschdorfer L, Negreiros WM, Gallucci GO, Hamilton A. Comparison of the accuracy of implants placed with CAD-CAM surgical templates manufactured with various 3D printers: an in vitro study. J Prosthet Dent. 2020. pii:S0022-3913(20)30235-3.

19. Henprasert P, Dawson DV, El-Kerdani T, Song X, Couso-Queiruga E, Holloway JA. Comparison of the accuracy of implant position using surgical guides fabricated by additive and subtractive techniques. J Prosthodont. 2020;29:534.

20. Al Yafi F, Camenisch B, Al-Sabbagh M. Is digital guided implant surgery accurate and reliable? Dent Clin N Am. 2019;63(3):381–97.

21. Verhamme LM, Meijer GJ, Bergé SJ, Soehardi RA, Xi T, de Haan AF, et al. An accuracy study of computer-planned im- plant placement in the augmented maxilla using mucosa-supported surgical templates. Clin Implant Dent Relat Res. 2015;17(6):1154–63.

22. Verhamme LM, Meijer GJ, Boumans T, de Haan AF, Bergé SJ, Maal TJ. A clinically relevant accuracy study of computer- planned implant placement in the edentulous maxilla using mucosa- supported surgical templates. Clin Implant Dent Relat Res. 2018;17(2):343–52.

23. Verhamme LM, Meijer GJ, Soehardi A, Bergé SJ, Xi T, Maal TJ. An accuracy study of computer-planned implant placement in the augmented maxilla using osteosynthesis screws. Int J Oral Maxillofac Surg. 2017;46(4):511–7.

24. Nickenig HJ, Eitner S. An alternative method to match planned and achieved positions of implants, after virtual planning using cone-beam CT data and surgical guide templates--a method reducing patient radiation exposure (part I). J Craniomaxillofac Surg. 2010;38(6):436–40.

25. Koop R, Vercruyssen M, Vermeulen K, Quirynen M. Tolerance within the sleeve inserts of different surgical guides for guided implant surgery. Clin Oral Implants Res. 2013;24(6):630–4.

26. Schneider D, Schober F, Grohmann P, Hammerle CH, Jung RE. In-vitro evaluation of the tolerance of surgical instruments in templates for computer-assisted guided implantology produced by 3-D printing. Clin Oral Implants Res. 2015;26(3):320–5.

27. Schnutenhaus S, Edelmann C, Rudolph H, Luthardt RG. Retrospective study to determine the accuracy of template-guided implant placement using a novel nonradiologic evaluation method. Oral Surg Oral Med Oral Pathol Oral Radiol. 2016;121(4):e72–9.

Implant Navigation System: Dynamic Guided Surgery

7

Luigi V. Stefanelli and Silvia La Rosa

7.1 Introduction

Dynamic surgical navigation (DSN) is a computer-guided free-hand technology that allows for highly accurate procedures in real time through instruments motion tracking, eliminating the need of computer-generated stereolithographic guides (static), and direct visualization. Dynamic surgical navigation works much like a global positioning system assisting the clinician in obtaining high levels of surgical accuracy during the execution of all implant surgical procedures. In this chapter, general considerations, workflow, advantages, challenges, emerging applications as well as clinical cases will be reviewed.

7.2 Implant Navigation System

7.2.1 General Considerations

Computer assisted implant surgery (CAIS) facilitates dental implant placement. It encompasses both virtual planning, with the aid of a specific software, and the use of a surgical guide [1]. Due

to its many advantages, including possibility of performing a flapless surgery, reduced surgical time and patient morbidity, this surgical technique has been embraced by clinicians across the world. CAIS is a prosthetically driven modality where prosthetic outcome goals determine surgical requirements of the case. With such integration between prosthetics and surgery, the best possible aesthetic and functional results can be achieved. In addition, regional anatomy is clearly visualized prior to surgery, so potential for iatrogenic injury can be reduced. This concept is known as "Prosthetic Guided Implantology".

There are two CAIS methods available today: static (sCAIS) and dynamic (dCAIS).

sCAI is based on the usage of a surgical guide that could be 3D printed, using additive manufacturing (stereolithography), or drilled, using subtractive manufacturing (numeric controlled machining) [2].

The "static" (sCAIS) guide is a computer manufactured appliance generated based on an implant placed within a CAD software. A drawback of this process is the inability to make changes once the stereolithographic guide has been fabricated [3].

The "dynamic" (dCAIS) option allows the surgeon freedom to make changes both during planning and surgery. In fact, dynamic techniques allow real-time visualization and verification of the surgical treatment [4, 5]. It is a computer-guided free-hand technology that eliminates the

L. V. Stefanelli (✉)
Private Practice, Rome, Italy

S. La Rosa
Private Practice, Sound Surgical Arts,
Tacoma and Gig Harbor, Washington, USA
e-mail: slarosa@soundsurgicalarts.com

© Springer Nature Switzerland AG 2021
J. M. Galante, N. A. Rubio (eds.), *Digital Dental Implantology*,
https://doi.org/10.1007/978-3-030-65947-9_7

need of computer-generated stereolithographic guides (static templates) and permits direct visualization.

There are two different types of navigation, optical and electromagnetic. In the Optical Navigation Systems (ONS), an optical position sensor camera tracks in real time the optically marked trackers attached to the patient and to the instrument you are using. In the medical field, ONS are used in otolaryngology, neurology, orthopedics, spine, interventional radiology, and maxillofacial surgery. Electromagnetic systems (EMS) are used in otolaryngology, interventional radiology, and neurology. In dentistry, ONS are the only type used. Currently, to the authors knowledge, seven optical systems are used in the dental field worldwide: Den X Image Guided Implantology System, Jerusalem; IGI by Image Navigation Ltd., New York; ImplaNav by Bresmedical Pty Ltd., Australia; Inliant by Inliant Dental Technologies, Vancouver, BC; Iris-Clinic by EPED, Taiwan; Navident by ClaroNav Technologies, Toronto, Ontario; and X-Guide by X-Nav Technologies, Lansdale, Pennsylvania.

Multiple studies have evaluated the accuracy of dynamic navigation systems. Gunkel [6], Siesseger [7], Eggers [8], and Wanschitz [9] reported an accuracy of 1–2 mm in vitro when using first-generation dynamic navigation systems.

Somogyi-Ganss et al. [10] used an early prototype of Navident, the system used by the authors in this chapter, to make 80 in vitro osteotomies. They reported 1.14 mm, 1.71 mm, and 2.99° for mean entry, apical and angular points, correspondingly. Wagner et al. [11] inserted 32 implants in 5 patients and reported an angular accuracy of 6.4°, with a range of 0.4–13.3°.

Garcia et al. [12] inserted in vitro 36 implants, 18 free-hand, and 18 by using a dynamic navigation system. They reported a significantly higher accuracy for all variables studied. Deviations using a dynamic navigation system were 1.29 mm at entry point 3D, 0.85 mm at entry point 2D, 1.32 mm at apex 3D, 0.88 mm at apex vertical and 1.6° as angular deviation; while using free-hand they reported a deviation of 1.5 mm at entry 3D, 1.26 mm at entry 2D, 2.26 mm at apex 3D,

0.57 mm at apex vertical, and 9.7° as angular deviation.

Block et al. [13] reported on the placement accuracy obtained by three surgeons using a second-generation navigation system (X-Guide, X-Nav Technologies) to treat 100 patients. The deviations were also compared with free-hand placement accuracy. Only partially edentulous cases were included, since a minimum of three adjacent teeth was required to hold a special clip enabling the navigation. The mean (SD) deviations with X-Guide were 0.87 (0.42) mm at entry (lateral/2D), 1.56 (0.69) mm at the apex (3D), and 3.62° (2.73°) angular. The unguided deviations had corresponding means (SD) of 1.15 (0.59) mm, 2.51 (0.86) mm, and 7.69° (4.92°). No statistically significant differences between individual surgeons were observed in the navigated placement.

Pellegrino et al. [14] treated 10 patients to whom 18 implants were placed using ImplaNav Navigational technology. They reported mean deviation values of 1.04 ± 0.47 mm at the entry point, 1.35 ± 0.56 mm at apex, 0.43 ± 0.34 mm of depth deviation, and 6.46 ± 3.95 degrees of angular deviation.

Stefanelli et al. [15] reported in a retrospective observational study on 231 implants (89 arches) using Navident (Claronav, Toronto) a mean (SD) deviation of 0.71(0.4) mm at the entry point, 1(0.49) mm at the apex, and a mean angular discrepancy of 2.26 (1.62) degrees.

7.2.2 Advantages of Dynamic Surgical Navigation

While both dynamic and static options currently appear to provide comparable in-vivo placement accuracy [1–3, 11–18], the dynamic approach provides the following advantages:

1. *Improved accuracy:* Dynamic Surgical Navigation (DSN) is more accurate when compared to free-hand implant surgery or free-hand guidance with computer-generated stereolithographic guides, as demonstrated in in-vivo publications. [13, 15].

2. *Eliminates the need for stereolithographic guides*: With all known advantages of the static surgical guides, limitations such as decreased vertical access in the posterior region remain a challenge. One of the greatest benefits of DSN over static guides is the ability to bypass this obstacle by allowing the clinician to navigate the drills at an angle that overcomes the given vertical limitation until adequate access is acquired, then correcting— in real time—the orientation of the drill to obtain implant ideal position. In narrow interdental spaces, like lower incisors, DSN surpasses static guidance as it is not restricted by the guiding sleeve sizes. Other drawbacks with static guides are the inability to change the plan within surgery, difficulty in obtaining proper irrigation to the implant drills, limited to no visibility of the surgical site, variable fit, increased cost and turnaround time.

3. *Software*: It is intuitive and easy to use.

4. *Versatile*: DSN is CBCT independent, therefore any DICOM file can be imported to be planned in its software. It is also implant system independent (any implant system can be used). The surgical plan can be changed three-dimensionally within surgery with minimum delay to the procedure. Intraoperative deviations from the predetermined surgical plan can be seen in real time by the operator, thus allowing for immediate corrections. DSN allows for direct visualization of the surgical field at any given time. Finally, DSN can be handpiece-independent. This is currently only true for one of the navigational technologies, Navident by ClaroNav. Being handpiece-independent provides great flexibility to the clinician. This is obtained by means of transferring an optically scanned drill tag to different devices such as either a high-speed or a low-speed handpiece, a piezoelectric device, and others.

5. *Real-time verification:* DSN allows for real-time verification of the restoratively driven implant osteotomies and implant placement.

6. *Real-time visualization*: DSN allows for real-time visualization of the surrounding anatomical structures. This is critical when we are navigating near the inferior alveolar nerve (IAN), the mental foramen, the maxillary sinuses, the pterygoid complex, and even in proximity to adjacent teeth or implants.

7. *Ergonomics*: The operator is not looking down and/or bending at the patient surgical site. Instead, clinician is looking straight at the computer screen in the navigational unit maintaining proper posture.

8. *Fiducial independence*: Although this is an advantage currently available only in one system (Navident by ClaroNav), being fiducial independent means the system uses high-contrast landmarks already existing in the patient (teeth, bone) instead of external fiducials that are embedded in a stent. Not needing to fabricate a preoperative stent and therefore being able to use one CBCT image to diagnose, plan, and perform surgery are the two greatest benefits of being fiducial independent.

7.2.3 System Design

Dynamic navigation systems are intended to assist preoperative planning and real-time positioning of tools during dental procedures when a pre-acquired CT scan of the jaw is available. In particular, they are designed to provide visual and acoustic real-time feedback on handpiece location and direction relative to a volumetric CT image and, when available, relative to a path planned on that image.

They are intended to be used by qualified dental surgeons as an optional aid in different dental procedures.

7.2.3.1 Principles of Operation

To guide drilling or cutting, the navigational system must accurately map the tooltip (working end of the tool) to a CT image of the jaw on which the treatment plan was prepared. It achieves this in three steps, as illustrated below (Fig. 7.1):

1. **Registration**: Computing a coordinate mapping between the jaw tracking marker and the coordinate system of the CT image so that the jaw and its image will be accurately aligned.

Fig. 7.1 The figure shows the three principles of operation (calibration, registration, and tracking) that the software makes for an accurate and dynamic navigated surgery (Navident by ClaroNav)

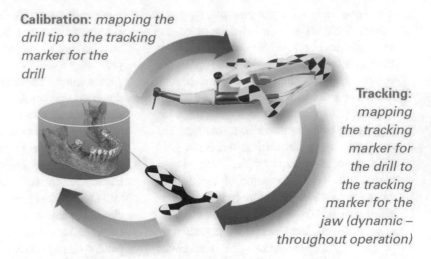

Calibration: *mapping the drill tip to the tracking marker for the drill*

Tracking: *mapping the tracking marker for the drill to the tracking marker for the jaw (dynamic – throughout operation)*

Registration: *mapping the tracking marker for the jaw to the CT image and planning the drill site*

2. **Calibration:** Measuring the location and orientation of the tooltip in the coordinate system, using an optical tracking marker attached to the handpiece driving the tool.
3. **Tracking:** Measuring the coordinate mapping between an optical tracking marker in the jaw and in the handpiece. This is dynamic and is done throughout the operation.

Registration

Registration is accomplished by computing a coordinate mapping that maximizes the degree of alignment between measured, or known, locations in the jaw markers (the "real world") and their appearance in the CT image. These locations can be defined by the known geometry of one or more artificial objects, generically called "fiducial markers", which are attached to the jaw prior to the CT scan. They can also be surface features, locations or shapes, that naturally appear with good contrast in any CT scan.

Calibration

Calibration of the tooltip is accomplished using a Calibrator tool. It carries an optical marker and a set of surface features with precisely known locations. The features are designed to be coupled with complementary surface features on the handpiece or tooltip, such as pins that fit into the handpiece

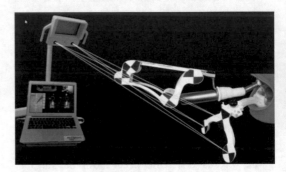

Fig. 7.2 The figure shows the triangulation between the two cameras, the handpiece and the jaw to be treated

chuck. Once the tool surface feature is pressed momentarily against the Calibrator surface feature, the location of the feature in the handpiece marker is established by mapping it from the known feature location in the calibrator marker coordinate system.

Tracking

The optical markers are printed or laser-etched on rigid parts called "tags," which are rigidly attached to the object they are tracking (jaw or handpiece). They are motion-tracked by a stereoscopic video camera (Fig. 7.2).

During surgery, the stereo video stream is sent to the computer, where the images are analyzed to detect, pinpoint and triangulate checkerboard optical targets to figure out their exact 3D location relative to the camera. The arrangement of the detected targets is then compared to known target arrangements in the markers to detect each pattern and compute its pose relative to the camera body. The mapping between the handpiece and jaw markers is computed by combining the measured poses of the individual markers.

7.2.4   Implant Placement Workflow

7.2.4.1 Dynamic Navigation with a Radiologic Stent

For all dental navigational technologies a radiographic stent/clip is required in both diagnostic and surgical phases.

This protocol, for partially edentulous patients, unfolds into four steps:

1. Stent / clip molding.
2. Scan.
3. Plan.
4. Place.

1. Stent
A thermoplastic material or clip is fixed on the residual teeth assuring there is no stent dislodgement while opening and closing the mouth.
2. Scan
A CBCT is obtained with the thermoplastic stent / clip in the patient mouth, affixed to a fiducial marker (Fig. 7.3). It is imperative that the stent is fitted in the exact same

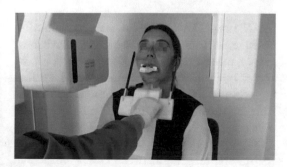

Fig. 7.3 CBCT with the radiographic stent fixed on the residual teeth

location, without movement, from fabrication to scanning and during implant surgery, to assure complete accuracy. An improperly fitted stent will lead to an inaccurate and unsafe navigation. Fabrication of a new stent is then required, adding unnecessary chair time for both patient and clinician.
3. Plan
The DICOM file from the CBCT is imported to the navigational software followed by the STL file from the virtual restorative plan. The implant planning is done through virtual libraries available within the software (direct wax-up) and/or through an STL file containing the ideal virtual restorative plan (indirect wax-up) (Fig. 7.4).
4. Place
To initiate the procedure, the clip/stent is placed in the patient mouth connected to a specific jaw tag. For most of technologies available, a specific handpiece is needed. Once the two are visible by the cameras, navigation may start.

Surgery starts with drill axis and tip calibration, followed by accuracy check on the calibration, to assure that measurements are close to the true value. This can be proved by assessing congruency between what the surgeon touches and what he can see on the computer screen (Fig. 7.5). The navigated osteotomies follow with instant guidance in the computer screen (see dynamic surgery below).

7.2.4.2 Dynamic Navigation with the Trace and Place Protocol

With the this technology, stent preparation is eliminated and workflow encompasses the following steps:

1. Scan.
2. Plan.
3. Trace and Place.

1. Scan: A diagnostic CBCT is obtained without a stent.

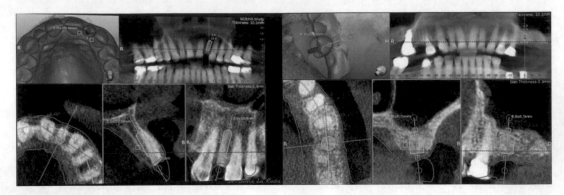

Fig. 7.4 Prosthetic driven implant planning

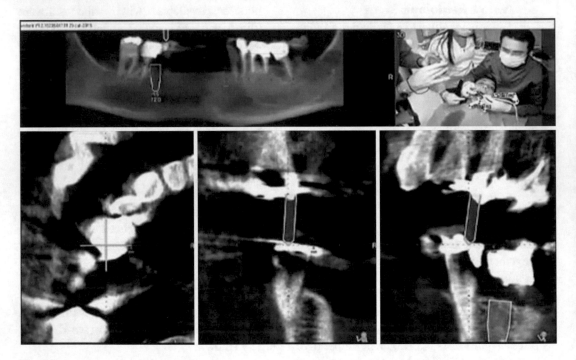

Fig. 7.5 Accuracy check before the surgery

2. Plan: Same protocol as planning with a stent above.
3. Trace Registration (TR)/Trace and Place (TaP).

Instead of external/artificial fiducials embedded in a radiographic stent, TR utilizes high-contrast landmarks that are visible on the CBCT image or a surface scan (STL) registered to it, such as teeth or abutments. The software requires 3–6 landmarks to be chosen for registration/alignment between the corresponding jaw and CBCT image. Unlike the fiducials on a fiducial-based registration (which have a fixed and known shape), the shape of these landmarks needs to be sensed by the DSN system prior to surgery utilizing a "Surface Contact Scan" approach. An optically trackable ball-tip tool is used to trace 100 points per chosen landmark, to be related to the CBCT by the computer software, thus providing registration mapping between CBCT image and the patient jaw (Fig. 7.6). The method described above is fiducial independent.

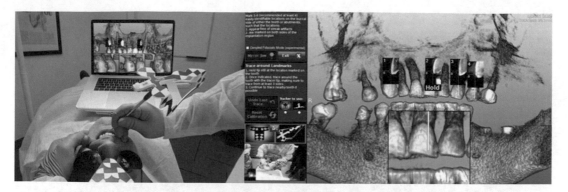

Fig. 7.6 Tracer used to trace the chosen landmarks/teeth as reference for the matching of the 3D mesh points with the equivalent on CBCT 3D rendering

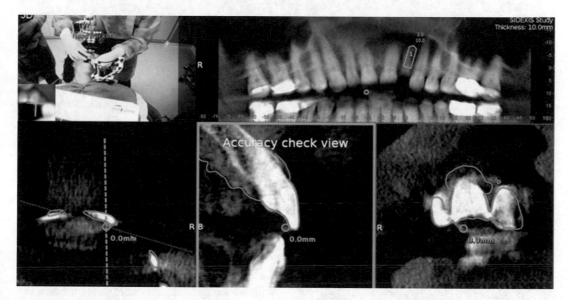

Fig. 7.7 Accuracy check of the trace registration

With TR technology (TaP) the workflow has been simplified by:

- Not needing to prepare a preoperative stent; hence, minimizing chair time to both patient and clinician. Developing a full digital workflow.
- The ability to use one CBCT image to diagnose, plan, and perform surgery. It is not only more streamlined, cost-effective and simpler, but also minimizes unnecessary radiation exposure to the patient.

Once the tracing is complete, software will prompt the clinician to the accuracy check screen to verify that measurements are close to the true value, to assure the accuracy and procedure safety (Fig. 7.7). Drill axis and tip calibration are carried out followed by the accuracy check of the calibration; recommended at each drill tip change.

Dynamic Surgery: Place

Once the accuracy check is verified, clinician may carry out the navigated osteotomies while verifying deviations with the planned osteotomy at entry, apical, and angular levels in the target view. Also, position of the drill during osteotomy in the coronal and sagittal views are visible (Fig. 7.8).

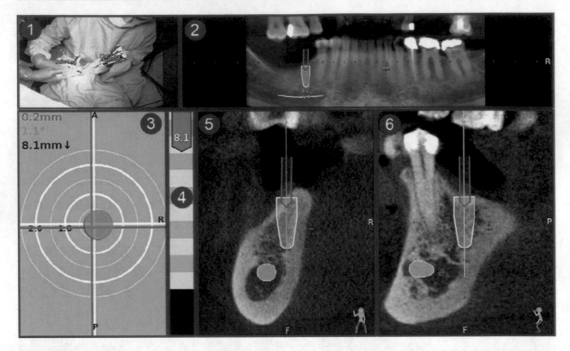

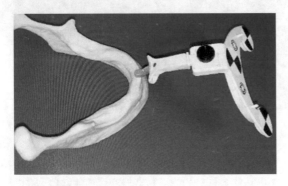

Fig. 7.8 The navigated drilling screen with all the views the clinician can see in real time during the surgery: (1) video stream, (2) panoramic view, (3) target view, (4) depth indicator/vertical distance to the planned implant, (5) coronal view, (6) tangential view

Fig. 7.9 Mini-implant for the totally edentulous patients

7.2.4.3 Fully Edentulous Patients

Treatment of the fully edentulous arches, or those in which residual teeth are not sufficient to provide a stable anchor to the radiological stent, requires the insertion of a mini-implant to which the radiological stent is connected prior to obtaining the CBCT image (Fig. 7.9). Another solution is placing rigid fixation screws in the respective jaw prior to CBCT image and using those as fiducials to register the jaw to the CBCT. From here, the steps are the same as for partially edentulous patients.

7.2.4.4 Surgical Accuracy Verification

With all navigational technologies, clinician can verify accuracy by exporting the plan as an STL and superimposing it with the follow-up CBCT image (Fig. 7.10).

7.3 Clinical Applications

With dynamic navigation, all implant surgical procedures can be completed. Given its accuracy, this technology has the potential to be used in orthognatic surgery, in the verification of bone pathology margins for its removal, and access of impacted teeth amongst others. Both navigated pterygoid implants and transcrestal sinus augmentation will be discussed.

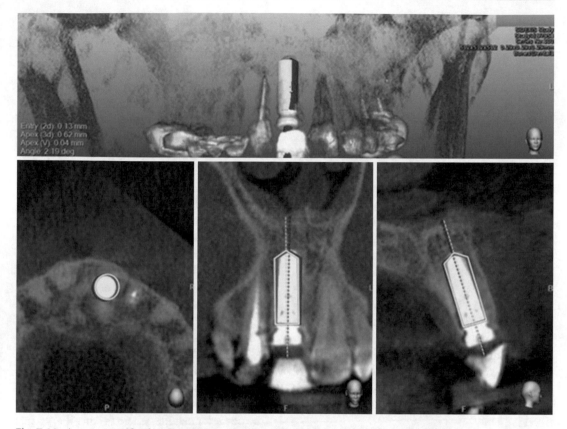

Fig. 7.10 Accuracy verification. EvaluNav application embedded into the Navident software demonstrating the deviations between the plan and the actual implant placement at the entry, apical, vertical, and angle

7.3.1   Dynamic Surgical Navigation and Pterygoid Implants

Dental implant placement in the posterior edentulous maxilla can be difficult due to inherent challenges to this particular anatomical area, such as restricted vertical access, limited vertical height of alveolar bone available for implant placement due to atrophy, poor insertion torque values and compromised long-term survival due to its inherently low bone density (typical D3–D4 type of bone) [19–22]. Limited vertical height can be solved by using short-body implants, doing sinus augmentation with immediate or delayed implants, placing implants in the pterygoid regions and, in selected cases, by the use of zygomatic implants [23–34].

The Glossary of Oral and Maxillofacial Implants (GOMI) defines the term of pterygoid implants as "implant placement through the max-

illary tuberosity and into the pterygoid plate." This definition is essential because, often, the term is mistakenly used as a synonym of tuberosity implant. The latter involves placement of an implant in the maxillary tuberosity and, sometimes, the pyramidal process of the palatine bone.

Understanding this difference is important because the area of maxillary tuberosity is composed prevalently by D3–D4 cancellous bone and the area of pyramidal process of the palatine bone and the pterygoid process of the sphenoid bone is composed by D1–D2 bone; it means that the success in terms of success rates in the short and long period of these two types of implants can be very different.

The use of pterygoid implants was introduced by Tulasne et al. [35, 36] at the end of the 1980s as a possible graft-less solution for implant placement in the posterior edentulous maxilla. It involves placement of one implant in the pterygoid region that is long enough to engage three different bones (the maxillary tuberosity, the pterygoid process of the palatine bone and the sphenoid bone). This particular anatomical singularity increases primary stability and implant long-term success.

Bone stress distribution values are influenced by different factors, such as bone quality, implant anatomy (diameter, length, macrostructure), implant position, implant-length to crown ratio and type of prosthetic device selected. Implant length does not seem to play a significant role in implant-bone stress distribution in bone qualities D1–D3. However, in bone quality type D4 (such as in the posterior edentulous maxilla), it appears to be an essential factor for implant success [37].

Although the use of pterygoid implants is demonstrated to be stable over time, this procedure is not widely used because of the need for a long implant (15–20 mm), which could cause potential damage to adjacent anatomical structures in a region filled with lots of anatomical variables. Finally, pterygoid implants share all the inherited prosthetic challenges of restoring a tilted implant.

The content of the pterygomaxillary fissure (PMF) includes terminal branches of the maxillary artery and the posterior superior alveolar nerve. Also, the content of the greater palatine canal (GPC) includes the descending palatine artery, vein, and greater and lesser palatine nerves. The ideal path of insertion of a pterygoid implant is from the maxillary tuberosity to the most apical point portion of the pterygoid apophysis, which is close to the PMF and GPC. The authors have measured this specific distance and reported to have a mean value of 22 mm. Cadaveric studies presented in the literature show that medium distance between PMF and GPC is 2.9 mm, with a minimum distance of 0.2 mm. This means that the use of implants shorter than the ideal length, with a safety distance of more than 2 mm, cannot be enough to avoid surgical complications.

Finally, literature reports that mean inclination of successfully inserted pterygoid implants with respect to the Frankfurt plane is 74 degrees in the anterior-posterior axis (sagittal view) and 81° in the bucco-palatal axis (frontal view) [38–42].

These angles demonstrate the level of clinical difficulty presented for adequate placement when using free-hand surgery.

The emergence of dynamic navigation systems (DNS) and its procured accuracy can simplify planning and facilitate the safe placement of pterygoid implants. The increased popularity of multiunit abutments (MUA) used in tilted implants can allow adequate prosthestic procedures in combination with pterygoid implants. This technique can become an alternative to either bone grafting or short-body implants in the posterior atrophic maxilla.

Dynamic navigation systems allow the clinician not only to perform a computer aided implant surgery, but also to check in real time if the ongoing surgery is accurate or not (Figs. 7.11, 7.12, 7.13, 7.14, 7.15 and 7.16).

7.3.2 Dynamic Surgical Navigation in Transcrestal Sinus Augmentation

In the posterior maxilla, where the maxillary sinus cavity is often atrophic, clinician may decide to either place a short-body implant, use a regular-size implant with simultaneous sinus augmentation, or do the antral augmentation with delayed implant placement. Transcrestal sinus augmentation is perhaps the most commonly used surgical technique for increasing the volume of the maxillary sinus simultaneously with implant placement where maxillary sinus atrophy is present.

Since Dr. Summers [43] published the osteotome-mediated technique in 1994, various techniques have been developed to access and elevate the sinus cavity. Main goal has been to eliminate the percussive forces of the mallet, therefore improving patient experience and minimizing potential drawbacks of osteotome-mediated technique, such as explosive forces to the maxillae with poor control, fracture or accidental displacement, membrane rupture, and paroxysmal vertigo. Many of these techniques use Piezo tips (PISE—Piezoelectric Internal Sinus Elevation) [44], or Piezo tips with internal irrigation (HPSIE—Hydrodynamic Piezoelectric

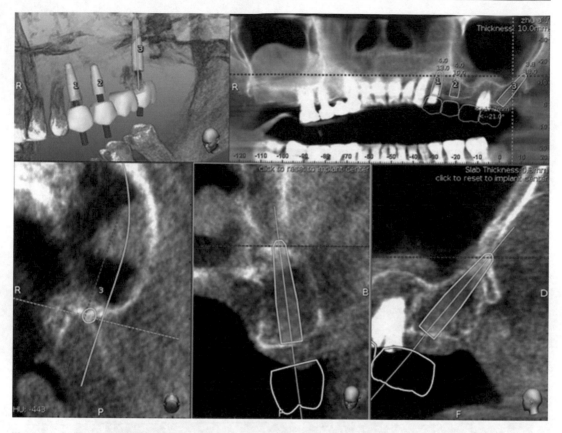

Fig. 7.11 Implant planning including a pterygoid implant

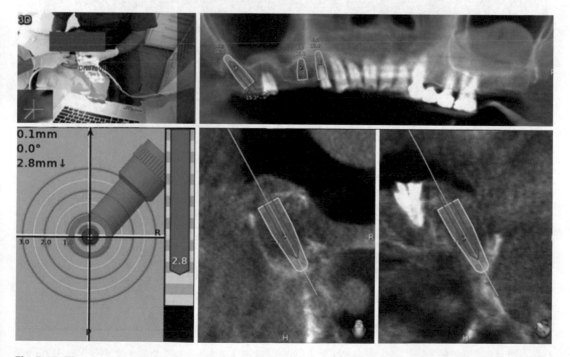

Fig. 7.12 The advancing of the drill during the pterygoid implant osteotomy

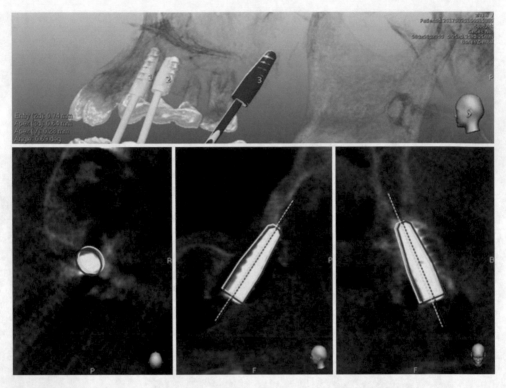

Fig. 7.13 Accuracy of the pterygoid implant. Deviations between the plan and the placement

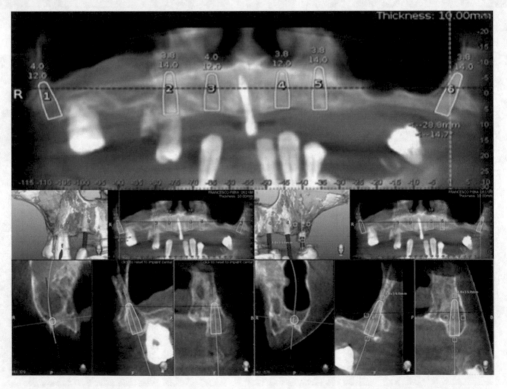

Fig. 7.14 Fully edentulous implant planning: four frontal implants and two pterygoid implants. The right three implants are placed free-hand and left three implants are inserted using a dynamic navigation system

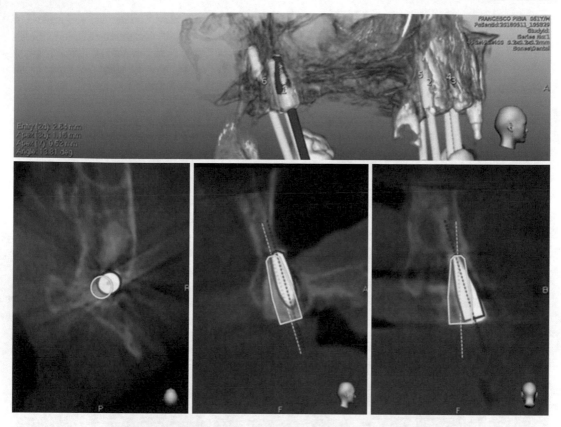

Fig. 7.15 Accuracy of the implant number 1 (right pterygoid) placed free-hand

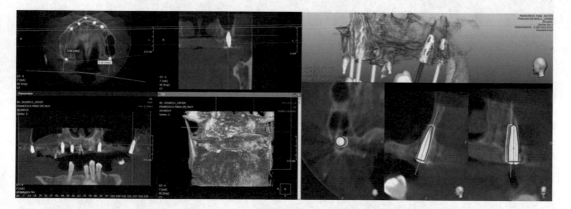

Fig. 7.16 Accuracy of the implant number 6 (left pterygoid) placed using a dynamic navigation system

Internal Sinus Elevation) [45], or Reamers (Hatch Reamer) [46], or burs (Densah Bur) [47] on a handpiece. All of these, including the osteotomes, can be combined with dynamic surgical navigational systems, becoming the perfect synergy to improve patient experience and accuracy of the procedures, while eliminating the need for guides or direct visualization.

7.3.2.1 Dynamic Surgical Navigation (DSN) in Transcrestal Sinus Augmentation (TSA) Workflow

Planning

To create an ideal restoratively driven plan, a CBCT and an intraoral surface scan (Fig. 7.17) are needed. The virtual plan is then exported as an STL file to the ONS software for planning purposes. Some navigational software programs also have virtual libraries, that can be used for planning when an intraoral surface scan is not available (only providing the alignment to the jaw curve, not the interocclusal relationship).

The DICOM file from the CBCT and the STL file with the restorative virtual plan are imported to the navigational software where the surgical planning is done (Fig. 7.18). Planning with the

transcrestal sinus elevation in mind (regardless of the technique used: Osseodensification, Hatch Reamer, or Osteotome-mediated), virtual implant is lined up 1 mm shy of the sinus floor in relation to the digital restoration.

Surgery

Patient is provided with an optically marked head or jaw tracker, which will be tracked by the micron tracker camera (optical position sensor camera) along with the drill tag throughout the procedure (Fig. 7.19). To register patient jaw to their CBCT, external fiducials are utilized on various navigational technologies requiring a stent. Using the TR, high-contrast landmarks already existing in patient teeth or fixation screws, allows for fast and easy registration. The accuracy of this step is critical for the accuracy of the navigation (Figs. 7.20

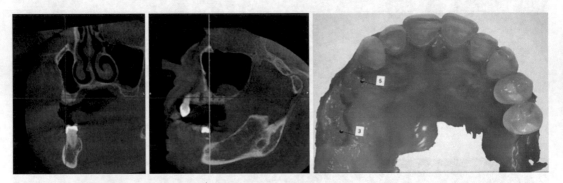

Fig. 7.17 Preoperative CBCT and intraoral surface scan. CBCT, demonstrating a mucous retention cyst

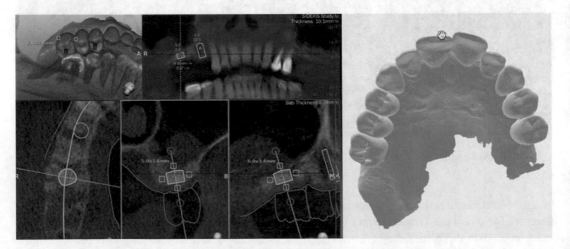

Fig. 7.18 Both the DICOM file and the STL file with the ideal virtual restorative plan are imported into the navigational software. The virtual implant is planned through the STL with the transcrestal sinus augmentation in mind

and 7.21). The drill access and the drill tip are calibrated to initiate the navigation (Fig. 7.22). Guided by the target view on the computer display, pilot

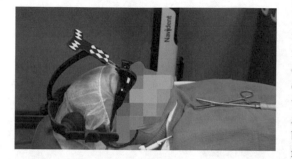

Fig. 7.19 Optically marked head tracker

drill is navigated to the plan length in real time (Fig. 7.23). Another feature is the ability to calibrate the width of the drill which can be seen virtually represented in real time (Fig. 7.24). In order to advance into the sinus floor, virtual length of the implant is increased by 1-mm increments allowing the lateral and apical compaction of the bone as a non-excavating technique, and the navigated delivery of a bone graft and the implant. It has been demonstrated that a bone graft is not needed in the transcrestal approach, especially when the RBH is 5 mm or greater [48, 49]. Condensation of the bone around the implant can be assessed with a radiograph (Fig. 7.25) and restoration is delivered as planned (Fig. 7.26).

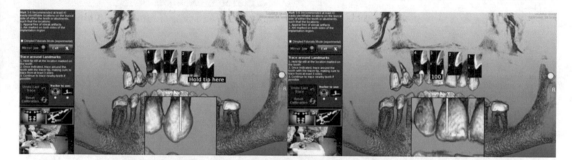

Fig. 7.20 After selecting landmarks for registration, 100 points per chosen landmark are traced

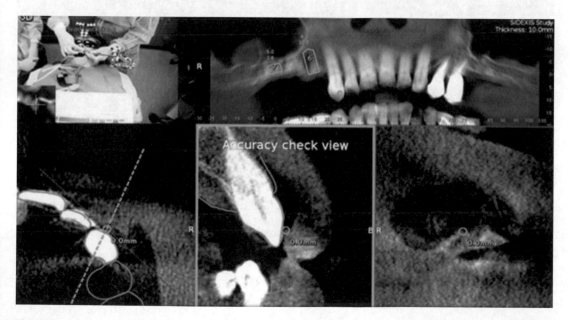

Fig. 7.21 Accuracy check of the trace registration

The endless possibilities to increase accuracy with dynamic surgical navigation should be considered; from Partial Extraction Therapy (PET), immediate implant placements, implants in the aesthetic zone, transcrestal sinus augmentation, pterygoid implants, zygomatic implants, apicoectomies, endodontic access of calcified canals, impacted canine exposures, Surgically Facilitated Orthodontic Therapy (SFOT), and ridge splitting.

7.3.3 Emerging Applications

As technology continues evolving, naturally, breakthroughs will occur. Some applications that are quickly advancing are listed below:

1. Fully digital workflow for completely edentulous cases.
2. Integration with pre-surgical CAD-CAM technology.
3. Control of rotational timing.
4. Surgical and non-surgical endodontics.

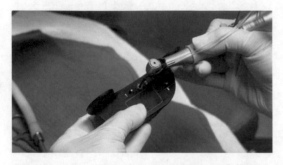

Fig. 7.22 Drill access and drill tip calibration

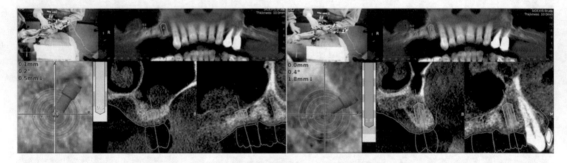

Fig. 7.23 Navigated osteotomies in the first molar and first bicuspid. It can be appreciated the real-time visualization of the sinus cavity and the canine

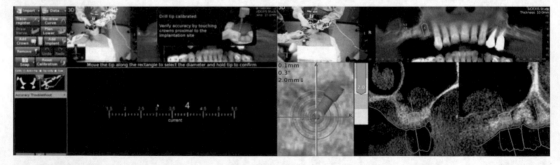

Fig. 7.24 Calibrating the width of the drills. It can be seen on the cross-sectional and tangential views the increased virtual width representations in real time

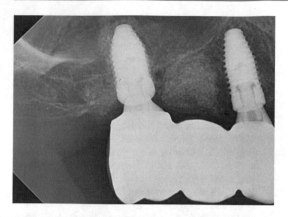

Fig. 7.25 Radiograph demonstrating bone augmentation

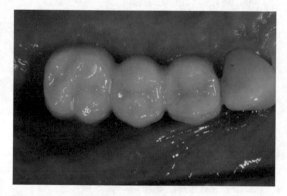

Fig. 7.26 Patient is restored with an implant supported bridge

advances simplifying its steps, learning curve becomes easier.

2. Mobile teeth cannot be used for registration. To overcome this challenge, it is recommended that teeth are splinted prior to acquiring the CBCT and performing surgery. In some cases, a block with embedded fiducals is available as an altenative to be used for registration.

3. Intraoperative periapical radiographs can be challenging if interfering with the position of the trackers. Placing the tracker in the opposing quadrant from the surgical site will alleviate this challenge. Another solution is the usage of a removable tracker.

4. Metal artifacts may interfere in the registration. In addition, registration can be done on the surface scan once both the DICOM and STL files have been registered to each other.

What is really important to define is that disregarding the technique used, clinician can successfully navigate any drill, reamer, osteotome, handpiecc, or piezo instrument to obtain a highly accurate restoratively driven implant placement. Dynamic navigation surgery, certainly improves accuracy of implant procedures when compared to free-hand protocols.

7.4 Challenges with their Solutions

As with any technique and technology, some challenges arise in the process of their utilization. Some of them can be listed below together with their solutions.

1. Learning Curve: Like with any procedure there is a learning curve. In the publication by Dr. Block and collaborators, it is suggested that after 20 cases are needed to become proficient [13]. Dr. Stefanelli and collaborators confirmed that accuracy significantly improved when comparing the first 50 cases to the second 50 cases [15]. This is based on the clinician skills and practice. In addition, as the technology

References

1. Tahmaseb A, Wu V, Wismeijer D, Coucke W, Evans C. The accuracy of static computer-aided implant surgery: a systematic review and meta- analysis. Clin Oral Implants Res. 2018 Oct;29(Suppl 16):416–35. https://doi.org/10.1111/clr.13346.

2. Cassetta M, Stefanelli LV, Giansanti M, Calasso S. Accuracy of implant placement with a stereolithographic surgical template. Int J Oral Maxillofac Implants. 2012;27(3):655–63.

3. Arisan V, Karabuda ZC, Ozdemir T. Accuracy of two stereolithographic guide systems for computer-aided implant placement: a computed tomography-based clinical comparative study. J Periodontol. 2010;81(1):43–51.

4. Berdougo M, Fortin T, Blanchet E, Isidori M, Bosson JL. Flapless implant surgery using an image-guided system. A 1- to 4-year retrospective multicenter comparative clinical study. Clin Implant Dent Relat Res. 2010;12(2):142–52.

5. Bornstein MM, Al Nawas B, Kuchler U, Tahmaseb A. Consensus statements and recommended clinical procedures regarding contemporary surgical and radiographic techniques in implant dentistry. Int J Oral Maxillofac Implants. 2013;29:79–82.

6. Gunkel AR, Freysinger W, Thumfart WF. Experience with various 3-dimensional navigation systems in head and neck surgery. ArchOtolaryngol Head Neck Surg. 2000;126(3):390–5.

7. Siessegger M, Mischkowski RA, Schneider BT, Krug B, Klesper B, Zöller JE. Image guided surgical navigation for removal of foreign bodies in the head and neck. J Craniomaxillofac Surg. 2001;29(6):321–5.

8. Eggers G, Haag C, Hassfeld S. Image-guided removal of foreign bodies. Br J Oral Maxillofac Surg. 2005;43(5):404–9.

9. Wanschitz F, Birkfellner W, Watzinger F, Schopper C, Patruta S, Kainberger F, Figl M, Kettenbach J, Bergmann H, Ewers R. Evaluation of accuracy of computer-aided intraoperative positioning of endosseous oral implants in the edentulous mandible. Clin Oral Implants Res. 2002;13(1):59–64.

10. Somogyi-Ganss E, Holmes HI, Jokstad A. Accuracy of a novel prototype dynamic computer-assisted surgery system. Clin Oral Implants Res. 2014;00:1–9. https://doi.org/10.1111/clr.12414.

11. Wagner A, Wanschitz F, Birkfellner W, Zauza K, Klug C, Schicho K, Kainberger F, Czerny C, Bergmann H, Ewers R. Computer-aided placement of endosseous oral implants in patients after ablative tumour surgery: assessment of accuracy. Clin Oral Implants Res. 2003;14(3):340–8.

12. Jorba-García A, Figueiredo R, González-Barnadas A, Camps-Font O, Valmaseda-Castellón E. Accuracy and the role of experience in dynamic computer guided dental implant surgery: an in-vitro study. Med Oral Patol Oral Cir Bucal. 2019;24(1):e76–83. https://doi.org/10.4317/medoral.22785.

13. Block M, Emery R, Lank K, Ryan J. Implant placement accuracy using dynamic navigation. Int J Oral Maxillofac Implants. 2017;32(1):92–9.

14. Pellegrino G, Taraschi V, Andrea Z, Ferri A, Marchetti C. Dynamic navigation: a prospective clinical trial to evaluate the accuracy of implant placement. Int J Comput Dent. 2019;22(2):139–47.

15. Stefanelli LV, DeGroot BS, Lipton DI, Mandelaris GA. Accuracy of a dynamic dental implant navigation system in a private practice. Int J Oral Maxillofac Implants. 2019;34(1):205–13. https://doi.org/10.11607/jomi.6966. Epub 2018 Dec 5.

16. D'haese J, Ackhurst J, Wismeijer D, De Bruyn H, Tahmaseb A. Current state of the art of computer-guided implant surgery. Periodontol 2000. 2017;73(1):121–33. Review. https://doi.org/10.1111/prd.12175.

17. Block MS, Emery RW, Cullum DR, Sheikh A. Implant placement is more accurate using dynamic navigation. J Oral Maxillofac Surg. 2017;75:1377–86.

18. Mandelaris GA, Stefanelli LV, DeGroot BS. Dynamic navigation for surgical implant placement: overview of technology, key concepts, and a case report dynamic navigation for surgical implant placement: overview of technology, key concepts, and a case report. Compend Contin Educ Dent. 2018;39(9):614–21; quiz 622, Review.

19. Sharan A, Madjiar D. Maxillary sinus pneumatization following extractions: a radiographic study. Int J Oral Maxillofac Implants. 2008;23(1):48–56.

20. Schropp L, Wenzel A, Kostopoulos L, Karring T. Bone healing and soft tissue contour changes following single-tooth extraction: a clinical and radiographic 12-month prospective study. Int J Periodontics Restor Dent. 2003;23(4):313–24.

21. Ellegaard B, Kolsen-Petersen J, Baelum V. Implant therapy involving maxillary sinus lift in periodontally compromised patients. Clin Oral Implants Res. 1997;8(4):305–15.

22. Branemark PI, Adell R, Albrektsson T, Lekholm U, Lindstrom J, Rockler B. An experimental and clinical study of osseointegrated implants penetrating the nasal cavity and maxillary sinus. J Oral Maxillofac Surg. 1984;42(8):497–505. https://doi.org/10.1016/0278-2391(84)90008-9.

23. Wallace SS, Froum SJ. Effect of maxillary sinus augmentation on the survival of endosseous dental implants. A systematic review. Ann Periodontol. 2003;8(1):328–43.

24. Del Fabbro M, Testori T, Francetti L, Weinstein R. Systematic review of survival rates for implants placed in the grafted maxillary sinus. Int J Periodontics Restor Dent. 2004;24(6):565–77.

25. Rose PS, Summers RB, Mellado JR, et al. Bone-added osteotome sinus floor elevation technique: multicenter retrospective report of consecutively treated patients. Int J Oral Maxillofac Implants. 1999;14(6):853–8.

26. Bahat O, Fontanessi RV. Efficacy of implant placement after bone grafting for three-dimensional reconstruction of the posterior jaw. Int J Periodontics Restor Dent. 2001;21(3):220–31.

27. Felice P, Barausse C, Pistilli R, Ippolito DR, Esposito M. Short implants versus longer implants in vertically augmented posterior mandibles: result at 8 years after loading from a randomized controlled trial. Eur J Oral Implantol. 2018;11(4):385–95.

28. Felice P, Barausse C, Pistilli V, Piattelli M, Ippolito DR, Esposito M. Posterior atrophic jaws rehabilitated with prostheses supported by 6 mm long × 4 mm wide implants or by longer implants in augmented bone. 3-year post-loading results from a randomized controlled trial. Eur J Oral Implantol. 2018;11(2):175–87.

29. Fan T, Li Y, Deng WW, Wu T, Zhang W. Short implants (5–8 mm) versus longer implants (>8 mm) with sinus lifting in atrophic posterior maxilla: a meta-analysis of RCTs. Clin Implant Dent Relat Res. 2017;19(1):207–15.

30. Anitua E, Flores J, Flores C, Alkhraisat MH. Long-term outcomes of immediate loading of short implants: a controlled retrospective cohort study. Int J Oral Maxillofac Implants. 2016;31(6):1360–6.
31. Bechara S, Kubilius R, Veronesi G, Pires JT, Shibli JA, Mangano FG. Short (6-mm) dental implants versus sinus floor elevation and placement of longer (≥10 mm) dental implants: a randomized controlled trial with a 3-year follow-up. Clin Oral Implants Res. 2017;28(9):1097–1107.
32. Chana H, Smith G, Bansal H, Zahra D. A retrospective cohort study of the survival rate of 88 zygomatic implants placed over an 18-year period. Int J Oral Maxillofac Implants. 2019;34(2):461–70.
33. Petrungaro PS, Kurtzman GM, Gonzales S, Villegas C. Zygomatic implants for the management of severe alveolar atrophy in the partial or completely edentulous maxilla. Compend Contin Educ Dent. 2018;39(9):636–45.
34. Davó R, Felice P, Pistilli R, Barausse C, Marti-Pages C, Ferrer-Fuertes A, Ippolito DR, Esposito M. Immediately loaded zygomatic implants vs conventional dental implants in augmented atrophic maxillae: 1-year post-loading results from a multicentre randomised controlled trial. Eur J Oral Implantol. 2018;11(2):145–61.
35. Tulasne JF. Implant treatment of missing posterior dentition. In: Albrektson T, Zarb G, editors. The Brånemark osseointegrated implant. Chicago: Quintessence; 1989. p. 103–58.
36. Tulasne JF. Osseointegrated fixtures in the pterygoid region. In: Worthington P, Brånemark PI, editors. Advanced osseointegration surgery, applications in the maxillofacial region. Chicago: Quintessence; 1992. p. 182–8.
37. Baggi L, Capelloni I, Di Girolamo M, Maceri F, Vairo G. The influence of implant diameter and length on stress distribution of osseointegrated implants related to crestal bone geometry: a three-dimensional finite element analysis. J Prosthet Dent. 2008;100(6):422–31.
38. Uchida Y, Yamashita Y, Danjo A, Shibata K, Kuraoka A. Computed tomography and anatomical measurements of critical sites for endosseous implants in the pterygomaxillary region: a cadaveric study. Int J Oral Maxillofac Surg. 2017;46(6):798–804.
39. Rodríguez X, Lucas-Taulé E, Elnayef B, Altuna P, Gargallo-Albiol J, Peñarrocha Diago M, Hernandez-Alfaro F. Anatomical and radiological approach to pterygoid implants: a cross-sectional study of 202 cone beam computed tomography examinations. Int J Oral Maxillofac Surg. 2016;45(5): 636–40.
40. Bidra AS, Huynh-Ba G. Implants in the pterygoid region: a systematic review of the literature. Int J Oral Maxillofac Surg. 2011;40(8):773–81.
41. Candel E, Peñarrocha D, Peñarrocha M. Rehabilitation of the atrophic posterior maxilla with pterygoid implants: a review. J Oral Implantol. 2012;38 spec no:461–6.
42. Araujo RZ, Santiago Júnior JF, Cardoso CL, Benites Condezo AF, Moreira Júnior R, Curi MM. Clinical outcomes of pterygoid implants: systematic review and meta-analysis. J Craniomaxillofac Surg. 2019;47(4):651–60.
43. Summers RB. Anew concept in maxillary implant surgery: the Osteotome technique. Compend Contin Educ Dent. 1994;15:152–8.
44. Sohn DS, Lee JS, An KM, Choi BJ. Piezoelectric Internal Sinus Elevation (PISE) technique: a new method for internal sinus elevation. Implant Dent. 2009;18:458–63.
45. Kim JM, Sohn DS, Bae MS, Moon JW, Lee JH, Park IS. Flapless transcrestal sinus augmentation using hydrodynamic piezoelectric internal sinus elevation with autologous concentrated growth factors alone. Implant Dent. 2014;23:168–74.
46. Ahn SH, Park EJ, Klm ES. Reamer-mediated transalveolar sinus floor elevation without osteotome and simultaneous implant placement in the maxillary molar area: clinical outcomes of 391 implants in 380 patients. Clin Oral Implants Res. 2012;23(7): 866–72.
47. Huwais S, Mazor Z, Ioannou A, Gluckman H, Neiva R. A multicenter retrospective clinical study with up-to-5-year follow-up utilizing a method that enhances bone density and allows for transcrestal sinus augmentation through compaction grafting. Int J Oral Maxillofac Implants. 2018;33:1305–11.
48. Del Fabbro M, Corbella S, Wenstein T, Ceresoli V, Taschieri S. Implant survival rate after osteotome mediated sinus augmentation: a systematic review. Clin Implant Dent. 2011;14(S1):e159.
49. Duan DH, Fu JH, Qi W, Du Y, Pan J, Wang HL. Graft-free maxillary sinus floor elevation: a systematic review and meta-analysis. J Periodontol. 2017;88(6):550–64.

Part III

Guided Bone Regeneration

Clinical Applications of Digital Technologies for Combined Regenerative Procedures

8

Jorge M. Galante

8.1 Introduction

It is the purpose of this chapter to demonstrate the benefits of modern technologies in daily practice and different combinations that can be applied to improve and facilitate complex procedures that dentistry faces every day.

It is described, from series of clinical cases, the application of digital principles for preparing the patient for implant therapy and planning regenerative procedures. Said applications range from simple mock-up design for the evaluation and definition of patient best treatment option, to guided surgical planning with simultaneous provisional manufacturing for immediate loading protocols. Also, the preparation of stereolithographic models, or even custom devices such as mini plates or meshes, which can enhance complex tridimensional bone regeneration cases.

8.2 Lab Evolution

For some time now, dental laboratories have become true *digital design* laboratories, where artisanal and manual work has been transformed into a very different task, since design is basically done through a software that allows different anatomies of prosthetic reconstructions to be applied on a screen, rather than on a plaster model (Fig. 8.1). For this purpose, said software programs have libraries with different tooth anatomies, shapes, and sizes that allow a very ideal approximation of the work to be done; not in artisanal form, but now in a digital way (Fig. 8.2).

As it was clearly described in Chap. 1, digital models can be obtained through scanning, either directly from the mouth of the patient by IOS, or in an indirect way through alginate or silicone impressions following EOS scanning, and then exported into a design software.

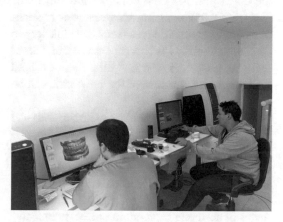

Fig. 8.1 Digital lab concept

J. M. Galante (✉)
Universidad de Buenos Aires,
Ciudad Autónoma de Buenos Aires, Argentina

© Springer Nature Switzerland AG 2021
J. M. Galante, N. A. Rubio (eds.), *Digital Dental Implantology*,
https://doi.org/10.1007/978-3-030-65947-9_8

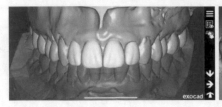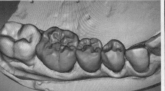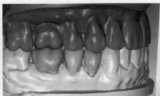

Fig. 8.2 Virtual tooth libraries

8.3 Case Series

Multiple applications of digital technology can be applied to diagnose and provide each patient a customized treatment plan that can be followed to increase accuracy and predictability. Focus on implant therapy and regenerative procedures is made in the following cases. However, infinite number of variables can be described for general dentistry.

8.3.1 Diagnosis and Development of Different Treatment Options

Next cases demonstrate that detailed virtual diagnostic can help improve clinical resources for the benefit of the patient.

8.3.1.1 Patient #1

This patient, who is missing the four incisors of the upper jaw, has bone collapse and soft tissue loss (Fig. 8.3a). A removable prosthesis replaces the missing teeth. The prosthesis has pink acrylic vestibular flank, which compensates for buccal collapse (Fig. 8.3b). When patient smiles, both white and pink portions of the prosthesis can be visualized (Fig. 8.3c).

One of the possibilities for assessing surgical planning consists in taking conventional impressions to obtain physical models that are then scanned and imported into a CAD software for waxing of the missing teeth. This design serves to perform different tests to appreciate the two forms of aesthetic expression: one of them incorporates teeth and gingiva, while the other involves only teeth (without pink structures).

Designs can be materialized either by subtraction methods (wax or PMMA milling) or additive methods (resin printing) to get an exact replica to perform a try-in and look for patient satisfaction (Fig. 8.4).

Once defined the prosthetic goal, an option can be performing a fixed hybrid prosthesis supported by two implants with immediate loading, or performing bone augmentation procedures and staged implant surgery.

Discussing with the patient said possibilities, a simplified protocol is selected by the means of guided surgery. Implant Studio ® (3Shape, Denmark) software is used for implant planning in sites 12 and 22 (Fig. 8.5). A resin template is printed and metal sleeves are attached to it (Fig. 8.6a). Guide fit is tested prior to surgery. In this particular case, temporary restoration is obtained by a combination of digital and analogue procedures, from the wax-up obtained in the diagnostic stage (milled PMMA) and then converted in the dental laboratory to a resin material following the traditional way (Fig. 8.6b, c).

Patient receives a fixed prosthesis on the day of surgery (Fig. 8.7). After 60 days of healing, implant integration is assessed and then, initial virtual design (preserved in a digital file) is used to design a monolithic restoration milled from a zirconia pre-sintered block (Fig. 8.8).

8.3.1.2 Patient #2

Patient #2 is referred for bilateral maxillary sinus elevation (MSE). Panoramic X-ray shows fully expanded maxillary sinuses, anatomy of bone ridges and deficient fixed prosthesis from teeth 13 to 22 (Fig. 8.9). In this case, treatment planning follows the vastly described digital flow: CBCT and STL files importation to a CAD software.

Treatment alternatives avoiding MSE are also evaluated, in concordance to patient requirements and risk factors assessment. Therefore, an implant spread protocol is evaluated. Digital

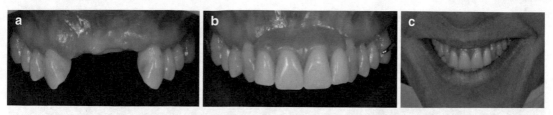

Fig. 8.3 Patient #1 initial situation (**a–c**)

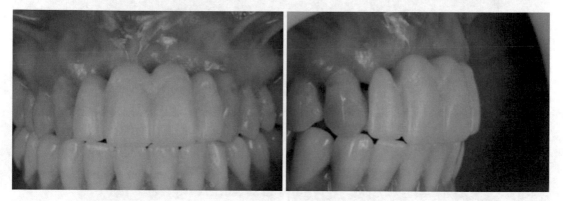

Fig. 8.4 Aesthetic assessment to evaluate the necessity of tissue augmentation

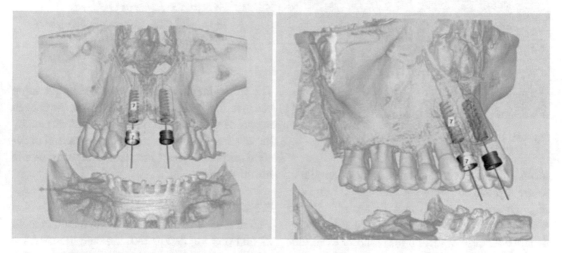

Fig. 8.5 Virtual implant planning

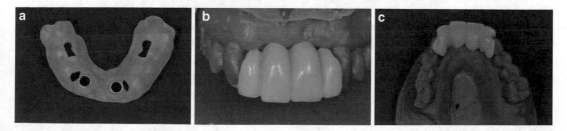

Fig. 8.6 Preparation for a guided immediate loading protocol (**a–c**)

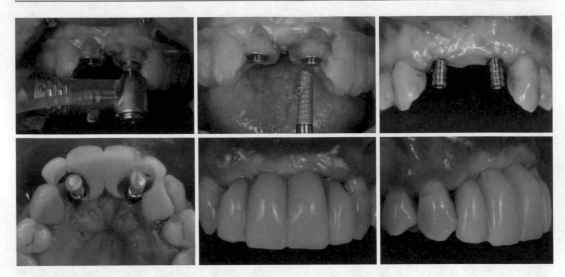

Fig. 8.7 Immediate loading of the interim prosthesis following guided implant surgery

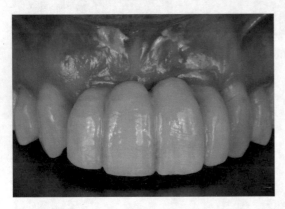

Fig. 8.8 Final zirconia restoration

tools allow for virtual distribution of implants to meet ideal positions for teeth 11, 21 and 13, 23. Moreover, sites 25 and 15 are planned to receive tilted implants, in a distal inclination, in order to emerge at second premolar or even first molar level. This implant orientation is parallel to the anterior wall of the maxillary sinus (Fig. 8.10).

Once planning is completed, a surgical guide is printed, to place SPI® (AlphaBioTec, Israel) implants in a guided way (Fig. 8.11a). Immediate loading protocol can be then planned to increase patient comfort, reduce risks, and save clinical time (Fig. 8.11b, c). Postoperative radiographic image serves as comparison for what was planned and what was achieved (Fig. 8.11d). Patient can

now complete treatment in a simpler, faster and more efficient way (Fig. 8.12).

8.3.2 Staged Surgery: Guided Implant Placement Following Analog Regenerative Procedures

The following cases show how virtual planning can get the most out of ridges that have been regenerated, to ensure proper amount of healthy tissue surrounding the implant and to avoid undesired pressure over grafted buccal walls while inserting the implant.

8.3.2.1 Patient #3

Patient number 3 presents a buccal fistula in tooth 21 and probing depths that indicate the need for extraction and bone structure compensation (Fig. 8.13a). Temporary restorations are also present in teeth 21 and 22. Panoramic X-ray reveals endodontic treatment of said teeth and CBCT shows periapical lesion of tooth 21. Bone defect appears to be wider than initially suspected and extension reaches tooth 22 (Figs. 8.13b, c).

First surgical stage consists in extraction of tooth 21 and guided bone regeneration (GBR) using xenograft biomaterials and absorbable membrane (Fig. 8.14). Tooth 22 is kept and

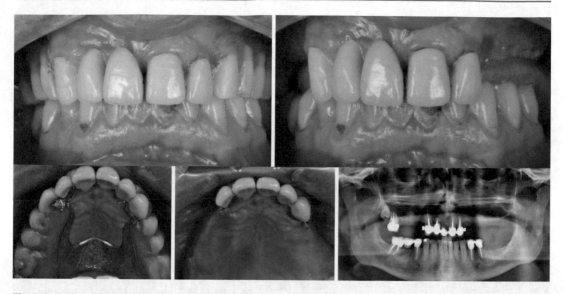

Fig. 8.9 Patient #2 initial situation

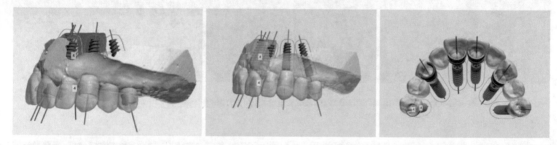

Fig. 8.10 Virtual implant planning of tilted implants and their emergence. Software visualization options permit implant assessment by transparency; removing the differ-ent textures, fading surface scans, CBCT, implants and restorations

serves as natural abutment for supporting a temporary fixed prosthesis.

Four months later, new CBCT is prescribed to be uploaded together with digital casts into a software used for guided surgery. Location of an SPI (AlphaBioTec®, Israel) implant is observed by transparency in the CBCT (Fig. 8.15a). As STL model is overlapped to the image, the gingival margin can be visualized to assess tridimensional implant location and thus, vestibulo-palatal, apico-coronal, and mesio-distal orientations can be perfectly established (Fig. 8.15b–d). Implant emergence is oriented to the cingulum of the tooth to be restored. With all these elements, a surgical guide is 3D printed (Fig. 8.16).

Second surgical stage consists in: performing an incision to fully expose the regenerated area

and, after template fitting, using an initial crestal bur followed by subsequent drills until reaching the desired diameter for the implant (Fig. 8.17a–c). It is very interesting to see the regeneration achieved, bone volume and quality. With the help of the surgical guide, implant is placed in the previously planned position (Fig. 8.17d).

A temporary abutment is used to adhere a resin prosthesis to shape the emergence profile (Fig. 8.18).

After a few months of healing, tissues show stability and thus, patient is ready for definitive restoration procedures (Fig. 8.19).

8.3.2.2 Patient #4

A step forward into GBR involves patient number 4, needing combined therapy of mini plate,

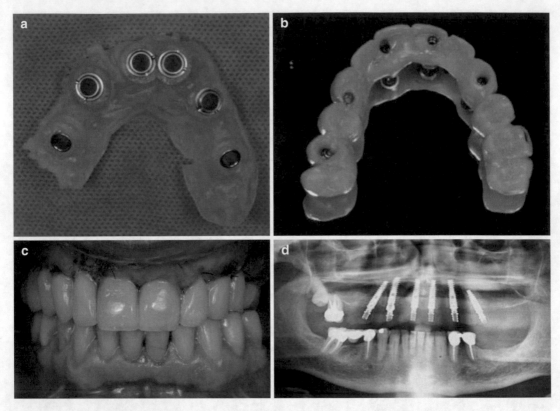

Fig. 8.11 Guided surgery for a fully edentulous patient using an immediate loading protocol (**a–d**)

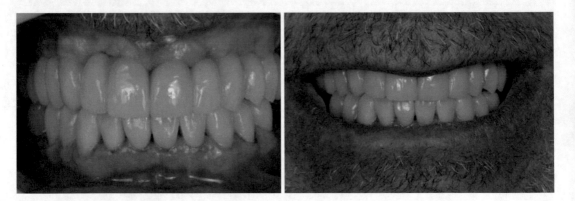

Fig. 8.12 Full-arch zirconia final restoration

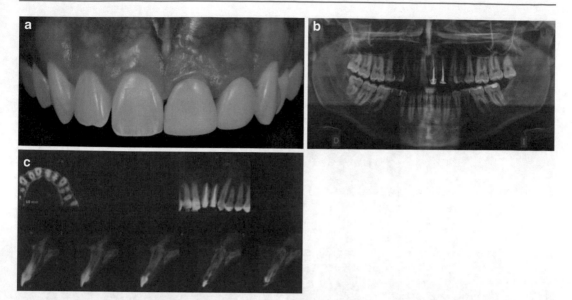

Fig. 8.13 Patient #3 initial situation (**a–c**)

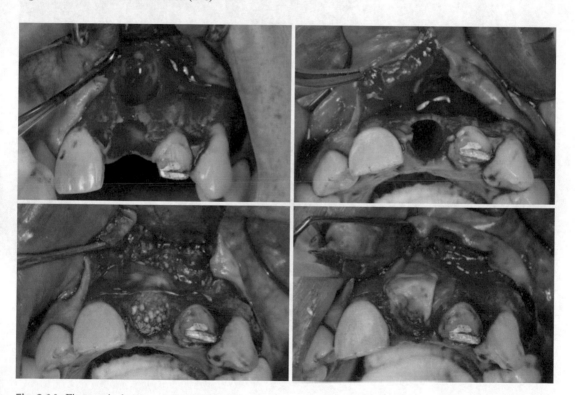

Fig. 8.14 First surgical stage

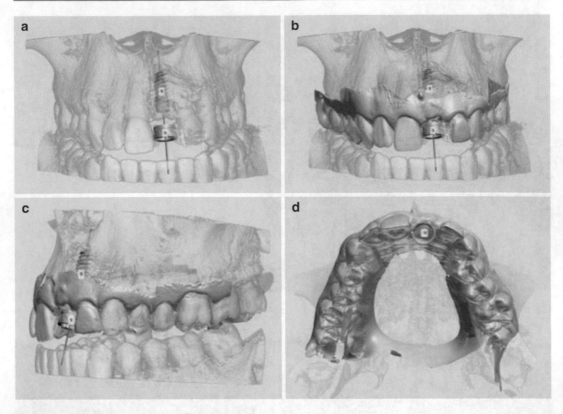

Fig. 8.15 Virtual implant planning of tooth 21 (**a–d**)

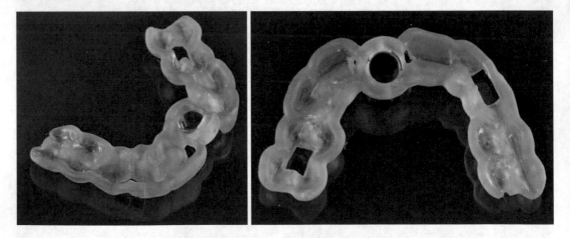

Fig. 8.16 Resin printed sleeved template

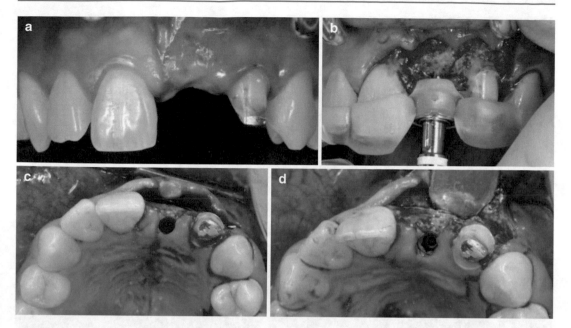

Fig. 8.17 Second surgical stage using a guided implant protocol (**a–d**)

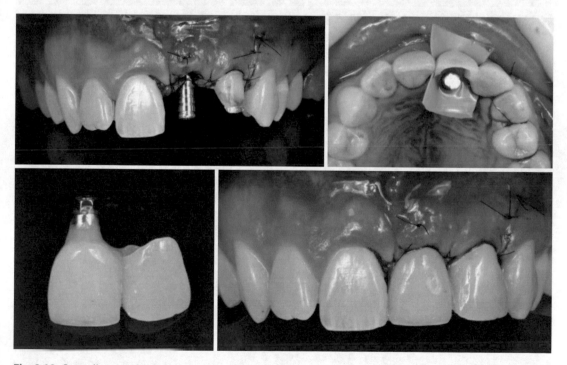

Fig. 8.18 Immediate provisorisation

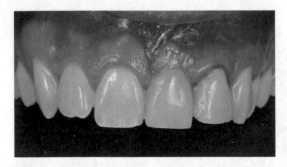

Fig. 8.19 Patient postoperative situation, ready for final rehabilitation

titanium mesh, and biomaterials (xenograft and pericardium membrane) to ensure appropriate tissue compartmentalisation and bone regeneration (Fig. 8.20). Teeth 12, 21, and 22 are missing in this patient and so, a conventional Digital Smile Design (DSD) is performed to establish functional and aesthetic parameters.

After healing period is completed, CBCT and digital casts are imported into an implant planning software. Best implant distribution and orientation can be defined by the means of guided surgery (Fig. 8.21).

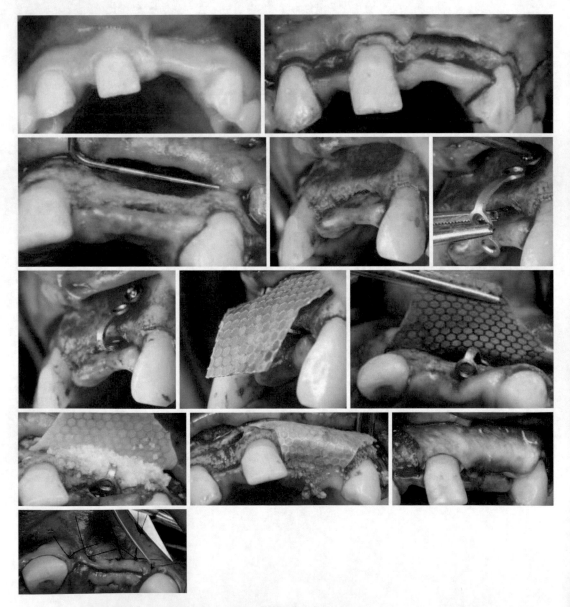

Fig. 8.20 Combined surgical approach for complex GBR procedures

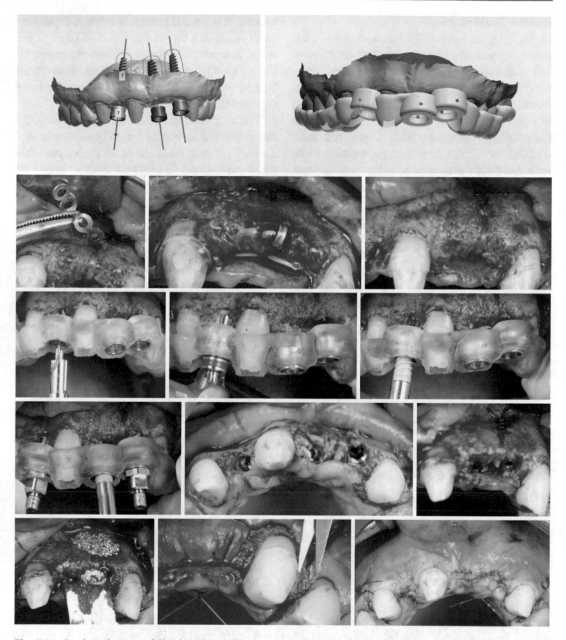

Fig. 8.21 Implant placement following virtual planning. Successful regeneration can be appreciated. Additional simultaneous grafting is performed and confirms virtual planning, which showed implant dehiscence at site 12

8.3.3   Staged Surgery: Stereolithographic Model from CBCT Rendering for Analog GBR Pre-surgical Planning

The following cases address the first option available since digital procedures were introduced for augmentation procedures. As described in Chap. 1, segmentation process from CBCT gives the clinician a valuable tool: a surface model that can be materialized. Commonly, these models are 3D printed and some of them can be steam sterilized. They allow for preparation of surgical tools, such as meshes and mini plates, in order to save clinical time and reduce patient morbidity.

8.3.3.1 Patient #5

In this case, the use of digital resources facilitates the realization of a complex bone reconstruction. The patient has lost the entire upper anterior sector (Fig. 8.22). There is a very poor clinical condition, where only tooth 23 (grade III of mobility) remains. Extraction is indicated in said tooth. The lower anterior antagonist sector is extruded. In an occlusal view, collapse of the premaxilla and volume deficiency can be noted. Stone casts were mounted in a semi-adjustable articulator in order to fabricate a temporary removable prosthesis.

CBCT exposes increased ridge resorption from site 13 to 24, severe loss of attachment in tooth 23 and presence of residual cyst from site 11 to 23. Treatment plan includes a staged surgical approach: first, extraction tooth 23, cyst enucleation and 3D bone reconstruction; and second, implant placement.

A bone replica is obtained by converting the DICOM file into an STL file and therefore, making a resin 3D printed model. A rigid titanium mesh can be prepared and adapted to the ridge contour in order to contain the biomaterial and serve as space maintainer. This structure tries to give clot stability for proper bone regeneration (Fig. 8.23).

The surgical approach exposes the entire anterior sector and shows the loss of bone support and the residual cyst, which involves almost the totality of the residual ridge (Fig. 8.24a).

Mesh adaptation within the printed model saves valuable surgical time, leaving sites prepared for micro-screws fixation, so that it can stay completely stable and movement-free (Fig. 8.24b, c).

An absorbable membrane is placed over this mesh and sutured to the base of the inner part of the flap to immobilize it (Fig. 8.24d). Subsequently, wound closure is performed in two planes to achieve primary closure. Also, the flap needs to be completely free of tension (Fig. 8.24e).

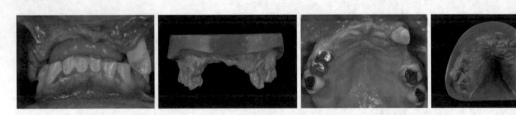

Fig. 8.22 Patient #4 initial situation

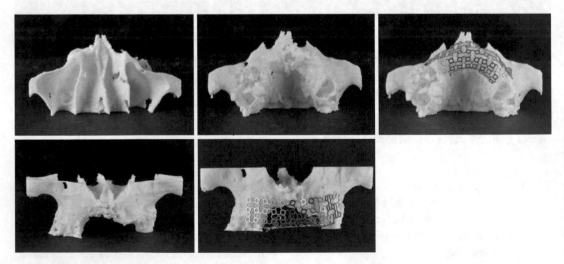

Fig. 8.23 Stereolithographic model of the maxilla for mesh adaptation prior to surgery. Once adapted, the mesh can be sterilized, saving valuable clinical time

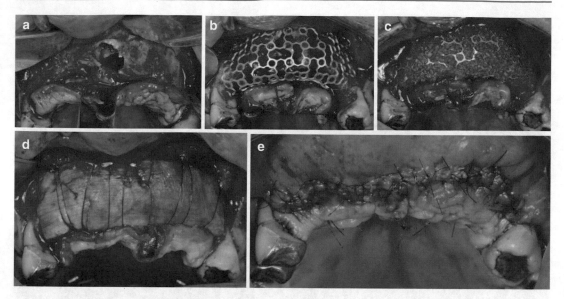

Fig. 8.24 First surgical stage for complex bone regeneration (a–e)

After 6 months, CBCT images show the mesh in situ and successful regeneration of the sector that was originally collapsed (Fig. 8.25). Implants are placed following conventional protocols (Fig. 8.26). Four months later, fixed partial hybrid prosthesis is performed by CAD/CAM technology and delivered to the patient (Fig. 8.27).

8.3.3.2 Patient #6

This is a case where a similar process is indicated (Fig. 8.28). In order to improve conventional GBR surgery, a resin 3D printed model is obtained from the CBCT. Both horizontal and vertical bone volume are insufficient to achieve implant stability and proper aesthetic outcome.

A titanium mini plate is previously adapted over the printed model to stablish a rigid vertical stopper, which contours and guides ridge desired anatomy. Once again, the possibility of having a pre-adapted mini plate in advance contributes to reduce patient morbidity and material contamination. In this particular case, the mesh comes embedded within a collagen membrane. Therefore, stereolithographic model is sterilized for mesh adaptation in a sterilized enviroment, immediately prior to surgery. Mini plates can be shaped previously and then sterilized for their use (Fig. 8.29).

The use of digital technology for these cases facilitates and decreases surgical time. Also, shaping of mini plates and/or titanium meshes tends to be more precise and easygoing than doing it intraorally; as surgical access, patient movement, presence of bleeding and saliva can complicate said procedures (Fig. 8.30).

8.3.4 Staged Surgery: Virtual GBR Planning and CAM of Surgical Materials

The following case represents a step forward into virtual planning, where not only the restoration and its aligned implant can be visualized, but also bone volume increment can be determined in order to fabricate mini plates and/or meshes to contain said desired volume. Materials can be produced either by subtractive or additive methods.

8.3.4.1 Patient #7

Patient #7 has lost his four upper Incisors due to chronic infection associated with endodontic failure. Extractions with simultaneous alveolar ridge preservation are performed. After several months of healing, a great volumetric loss of the entire

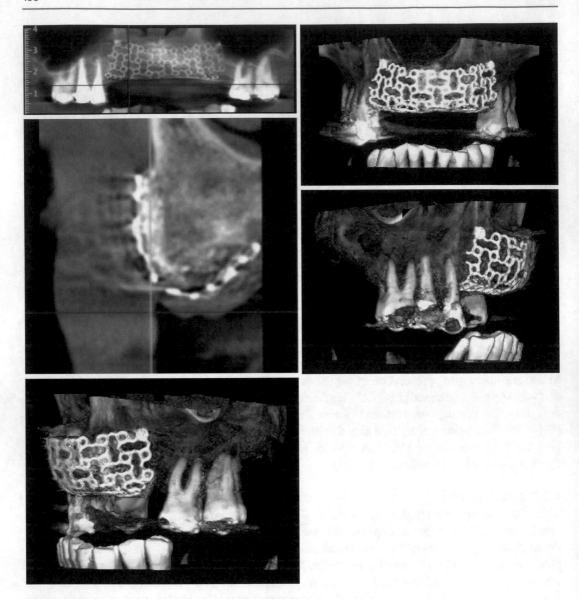

Fig. 8.25 Situation after 6 months healing (tomographic 3D reconstruction)

premaxilla area can be seen, together with very important horizontal and vertical deficit in the midline area (Fig. 8.31).

CBCT and digital models are imported into a CAD software, where an ideal bone volume simulation is planned. Over this tissue increment, a virtual mesh is designed to contain the future biomaterial in order to maintain that space and stabilize the clot. 3D reconstruction of the DICOM file is converted into a surface model (STL) and 3D printed using UV resin to obtain an accurate replica of the maxilla (Fig. 8.32a). Moreover, the virtual mesh is materialized by milling polyether ether ketone

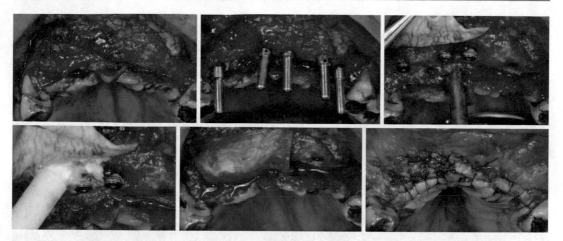

Fig. 8.26 Conventional implant placement and additional grafting at sites 11 and 21

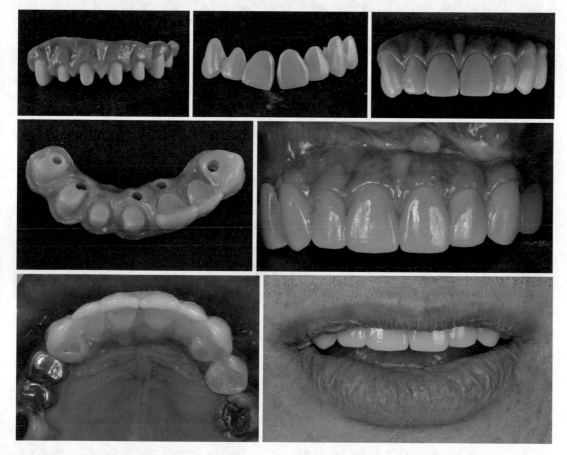

Fig. 8.27 CAD/CAM zirconia hybrid prosthesis

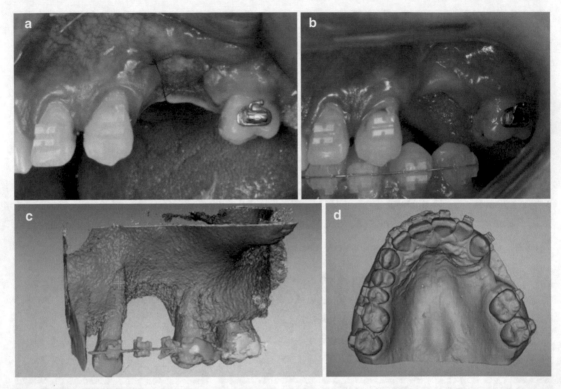

Fig. 8.28 Patient #6 initial situation (**a**) and soft tissue healing (**b**). CBCT reconstruction and STL files are used to perform a virtual planning and so, define a staged approach (**c, d**)

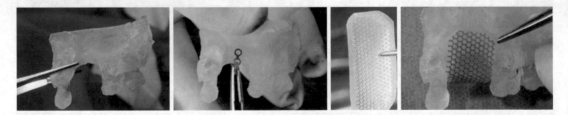

Fig. 8.29 Intra-surgical adaptation of the materials prior to incision making

(PEEK) material in a subtractive way (Fig. 8.32b, c). The 3D printed model of the maxilla serves to check adaptation of the milled mesh and simulate surgery. Therefore, it helps the surgeon anticipate possible complications that may arise during surgery and plan feasible solutions.

The surgical sequence shows the invaluable advantage of digital technology contribution to planning and execution of highly complex treatments (Figs. 8.33 and 8.34).

After healing time is completed, virtual planning is used to deliver guided implants following PEEK mesh recovery (Fig. 8.35).

8.3.5 Immediate Restoration Following Immediate Guided Implant Placement

Another example of the countless possibilities that these technologies offer to modern dentistry is virtual planning for combined approaches, such as immediate implant placement with simultaneous tissue augmentation and immediate restoration in the aesthetic area. Once guided surgery is planned, restorative procedures can be done virtually in order to print or mill the temporary prosthesis prior to surgery; also it can be fabricated manually by surgical simulation on patient casts.

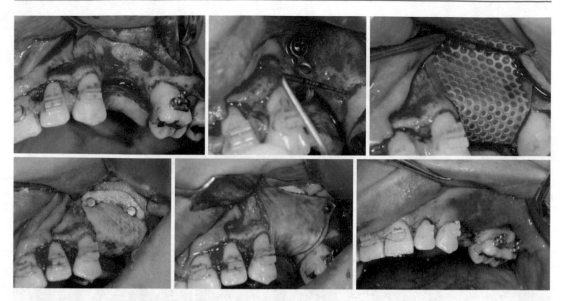

Fig. 8.30 Intraoral fixation of pre-shaped materials for GBR

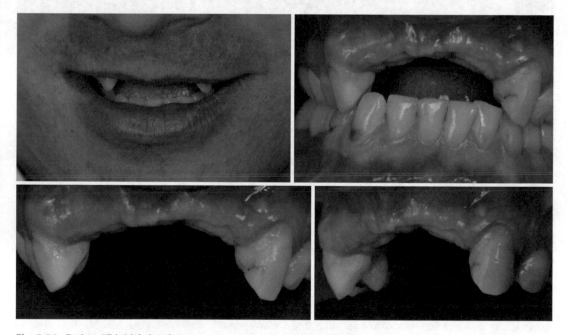

Fig. 8.31 Patient #7 initial situation

8.3.5.1 Patient #8

For this particular patient, a valid alternative to replace full digital workflow is described. Implant location is transferred to a model using the surgical template obtained from virtual planning, attaching an analog to the implant driver (Fig. 8.36). Thus, postoperative situation can be estimated to manually fabricate a temporary crown. Nevertheless, to improve seating of the abutment and overall prosthesis passive fit, abutment bonding to the restoration should be done clinically after surgical procedure is finalized.

Moreover, this procedure can be also done for CAD/CAM restorative procedures where surgical

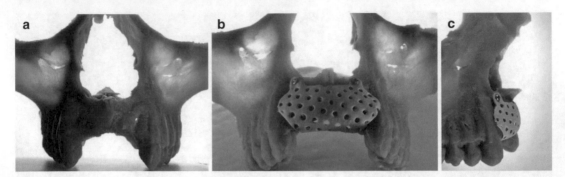

Fig. 8.32 Stereolithographic model obtained from CBCT rendering (**a**) and bio-compatible PEEK mesh obtained from a block milling process (**b, c**)

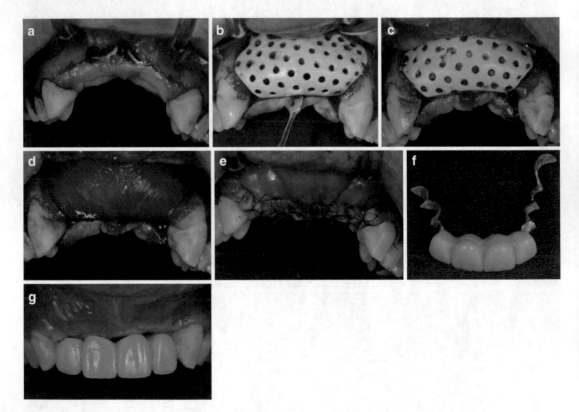

Fig. 8.33 Surgical procedure includes buccal-shifted incision, full thickness flap, biomaterial insertion, and mesh fixation (**a–c**). Pericardium membrane is used for coverage and free-tension closure is performed (**d, e**). Fixed temporary prosthesis is mandatory in these cases to avoid pressure over the healing area (**f**). Postoperative situation at 1 month time can be observed (**g**)

and prosthetic software programs do not share compatibility and so, do not allow file export/import between them (see Sect. 2.2.2, Chap. 2). In this case, a scan body can be attached to the analog placed in the model to re-scan it and allow for virtual design of the restoration (Fig. 8.37).

8.3.6 Virtual Outcome Assessment

Last but not least, superimposition of digital casts (surface scans) or CBCT renderings contributes to objective outcome assessment whenever measuring volume changes. Academic, research or

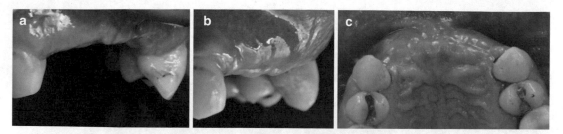

Fig. 8.34 Initial situation (**a**) and 6 months follow-up situation (**b, c**) shows successful volume increment

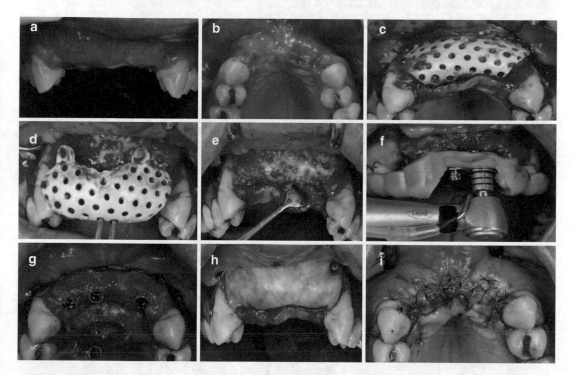

Fig. 8.35 Ridge volume increment can be denoted after healing period is completed (**a, b**). A full thickness flap is raised in order to recover the PEEK mesh (**c, d**). Bone augmentation is successfully achieved (**e**) and implant placement is done by the means of a sleeved surgical template (**f**). Complimentary guided bone regeneration is performed to optimize coronal peri-implant tissue (**g**) using an absorbable membrane (**h**) and ensuring a free-tension flap closure (**i**)

even clinical applications can be deduced from this valuable tool. Moreover, there is no doubt that virtual outcome assessment has positively influenced the way research projects are conducted nowadays.

8.3.6.1 Patient #9

Qualitative and quantitative precise outcome measurements can be done in this case by comparing pre and postoperative digital models after regenerative procedures are performed.

In this case tooth 21 has to be extracted due to root fracture. Concomitant multiple gingival recessions can be observed in the four upper incisors (Fig. 8.38a). Treatment plan includes a combined approach of immediate implant placement, GBR, and root coverage using a coronally advanced flap (Fig. 8.38b, c). Also, tooth 21 receives an immediate restoration (Fig. 8.38c, d). After a 6 months healing period, tissue appears stable (Fig. 8.38e) and so, final restoration is prepared using CAD/CAM technology. Digital measurements of initial

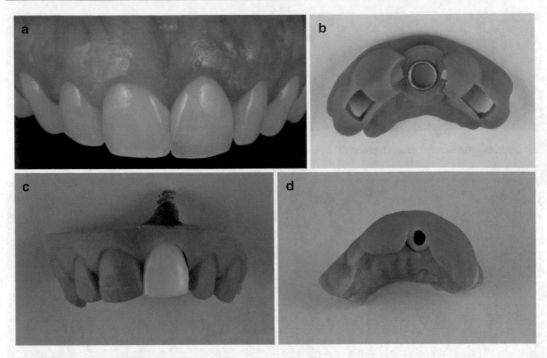

Fig. 8.36 Patient #8 initial situation (**a**), template fabrication by means of 3D printing (**b**), and temporary crown manual fabrication (**c**). Additional positioning device is designed to transfer restoration desired position (**d**)

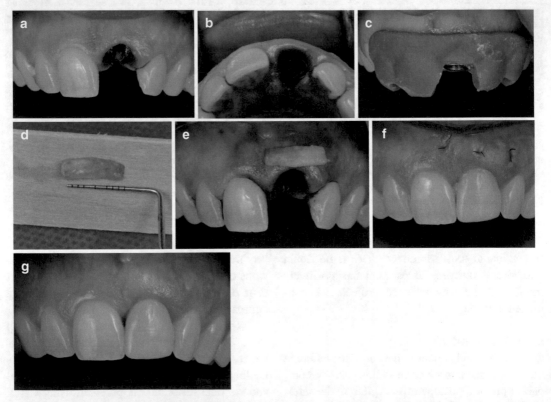

Fig. 8.37 Implant guided insertion following root extraction (**a–c**). Soft tissue graft is harvested from the palate to compensate for future collapse (**d–f**). Temporary crown enhances tissue healing and provide for optimum soft tissue contouring (**g**)

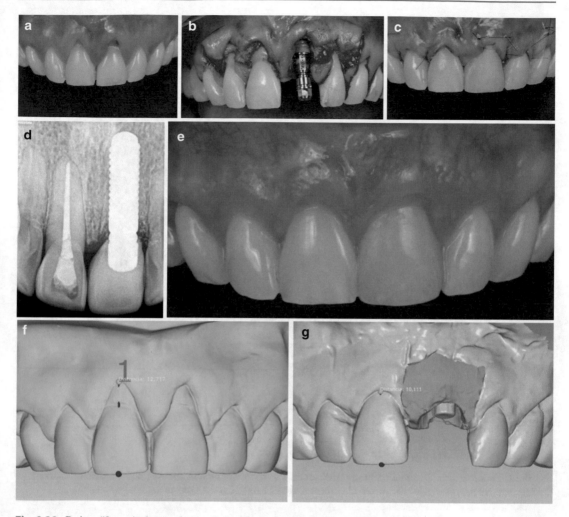

Fig. 8.38 Patient #9 surgical procedure and virtual postoperative outcome assessment (**a–g**)

and final situations are compared (Fig. 8.38f, g). Complete root coverage can be then assessed and gingival height reveals the amount of tissue gain and gingival coronal displacement.

8.3.6.2 Patient #10

In this other situation, a patient receives tridimensional bone regenerative treatment of the upper anterior area to compensate for important collapse and tissue loss. Titanium reinforced non-absorbable membrane is used as a barrier for the GBR procedure to contain biomaterial. A complete clinical sequence is shown in Fig. 8.39.

Once healing is completed, situation is analyzed using scans superimposition processes (Fig. 8.40). An objective evaluation can be made to assess qualitive and quantitive results. In addition, this can also be evaluated using CBCT rendering comparison (Fig. 8.39c, h).

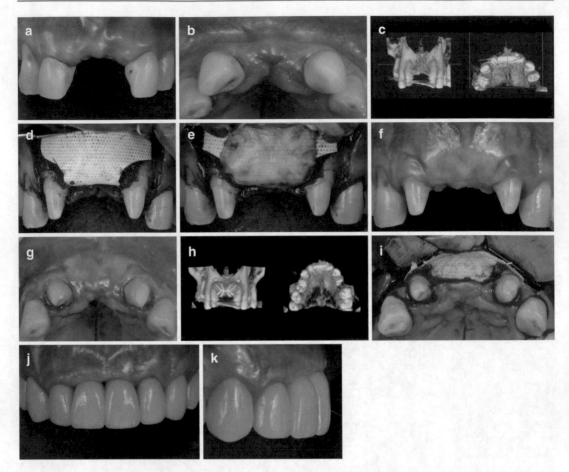

Fig. 8.39 Patient #10 initial situation (**a–c**). GBR procedure (**d, e**). Six months follow-up (**f–h**). Clinical outcome of the regenerative treatment prior to implant placement at sites 11 and 21 (**i**) and prosthetic final outcome (**j, k**)

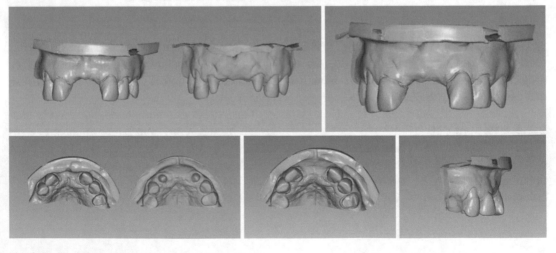

Fig. 8.40 Virtual assessment for volume increment

Digital Reconstructive Surgery

9

Luca Barbera, Niccolo Barbera, Alessandra Puccio,
Emanuele Barbera, and Marco Rossoni

9.1 Introduction

Talking about digital flows in modern oral reconstructive surgery does not mean rewriting traditional dictates of bone and mucogingival regenerative/repairing techniques. It simply means readjusting the classic schemes used in clinical practice to digital workflows, which are more channeled to follow a specific pathway, compared to traditional analog ones. That is, they require knowledge of a sequence of basic actions: starting from data acquisition, through design and finally, production of what is necessary (CAI-CAD-CAM Concept).

Another major change comes with greater integration of tasks performed by clinicians and technicians, who interact by exchanging and working, no longer on physical materials, but on files, especially during rehabilitation initial stages. In fact, to get the most out of the digital flow, emphasis must be given to data acquisition. This should be assessed before the beginning of following steps.

L. Barbera (✉)
Digital Dentistry Tutor, Monza, Italy

N. Barbera
University of Geneva, Geneva, Switzerland

A. Puccio · E. Barbera
Faculty of Dentistry, Digital Dentistry, Milan, Italy

M. Rossoni
Lab Odt ROSSONi e CASIRATI,
Treviglio, Bergamo, Italy

Moving forward to the design phase, working areas such as prosthodontics, periodontics, and implants need to coexist and interrelate to achieve functional and aesthetic outcomes.

Therefore, digital reconstructive surgery stands for standardization of pre-clinical processes to diagnose, design, and manufacture different elements, such as biomaterials or scaffolds, to enhance surgical stages that complement implant rehabilitation, saving time and reducing patient morbidity.

9.2 Biology of Bone Grafting. Current Concepts

As clinical and research work in the field of implantology evolves, soft and hard tissue preservation/regeneration concepts become inseparable. Therefore, they tend to fit into a single chapter, where peri-implant tissue support is strongly related to prosthetic structures. This introduces the current concept of "implant supported perio-restorative" unit (or apparatus), where each of its components must be optimized to meet anatomical and architectural characteristics of the others (Fig. 9.1). It is precisely in the concept of "architectural optimization" in which all regenerative techniques are based on, applied both to hard and soft tissues (Fig. 9.2).

This approach responds well to the needs of predictability and stability of results; not only

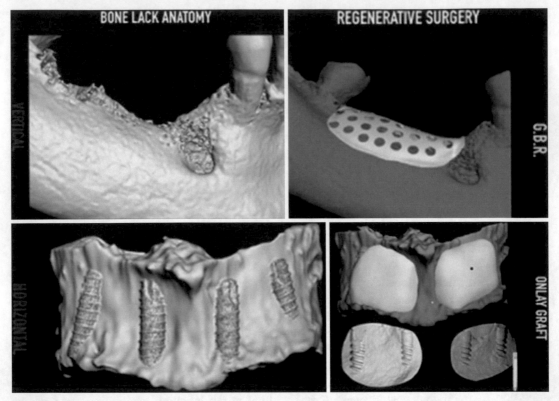

Fig. 9.1 Digital methods allow to clearly view information related to bone anatomy and contextualize it within a diagnosis and a therapeutic plan. Digital technologies facilitate titanium meshes design for guided bone regeneration and custom blocks preparation for onlay block techniques

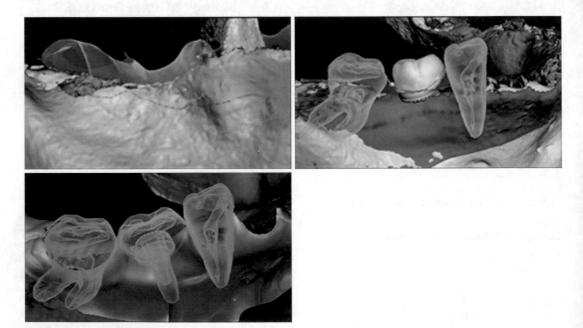

Fig. 9.2 Images superimposition relating dental, gingival, and bone renders to assess patient situation

functional, but also aesthetically, a fundamental requirement to date in terms of patient satisfaction [1–3] (Fig. 9.2).

9.2.1   Basic Concepts

The foundations on which most modern regenerative techniques are based on are three:

– Definition of an ideal architectural standard, attributed to the implant-perio-prosthetic unit, in terms of bone and mucosal support [3, 4].
– Classification of bone and gingival defects [5, 6].
– Biology of hard and soft tissue regeneration [7, 8].

There is a gold standard related to peri-implant hard and soft tissues, which defines the best possible condition for implant restoration survival, both from functional and aesthetic points of view. Peri-implant bone and peri-implant mucosa play a fundamental role on overall treatment prognosis. Thus, if an architectural rehabilitation of the peri-implant tissues is necessary, it must aim to achieve ideal conditions of said tissues. Furthermore, the starting clinical scenario (defect) and the desired result (correct tissue architecture) condition the operative choices in terms of regenerative surgery.

9.2.2   Reconstructive Parameters

Current trend and definition of ideal conditions for peri-implant tissue refer to the need for functional and aesthetic results. This explains the great emphasis and study dedicated to soft tissues. In his work, Deeb [4] summarizes the following conclusions regarding ideal reciprocal relationships in the "implant-abutment-gingival tissue-restoration" interface:

(a) **Periodontal phenotype:** *Thick,* with good availability of keratinized gingiva, interdental contact point situated in the middle third of the tooth and correlated with thick alveolar support and low tendency to resorption; *Thin,* with scarce presence of keratinized gingiva, contact point situated in the coronal

third of the tooth and correlated with thin alveolar bone with marked tendency to dehiscence and resorption.

(b) **Relationship between soft tissue and implant:** Implant should be positioned 3 mm apical to the gingival margin, at least 2 mm palatal from the buccal aspect, 1.5 mm from adjacent teeth, or 3 mm from another implant.

Additionally, Sonick [3] summarizes architectural foundations of bone support for peri-implant tissues. Ideal bone characteristics must always be comparable to those of a thick periodontal phenotype. Therefore, transformation of a thin biotype into a thick one before implant placement is pursued.

9.2.3   Biological Bases of Bone Regeneration

In this regard, it is considered fundamental:

– **Primary Wound Closure:** An appropriate design should consider volumetric increment to achieve a free-tension situation of the flap after suturing.
– **Angiogenesis**: This is one of the most difficult requirements to meet in regenerative surgery. When approaching reconstructions carried out with custom blocks of any nature, clinician must absolutely take into account vascular proliferation and blood imbibition which comes from the neighboring bone.
– **Space Maintenance:** Bone grafting has to have mechanical and dimensional stability as an essential prerequisite; that is, absolute lack of residual micro-movement.
– **Wound Stability**: Soft tissue micro-movement inhibits membrane barrier function by promoting epithelial migration to the site to be regenerated [3].

To translate all this into clinical-surgical practice, the decision-making flow regarding tissue rehabilitation comes as follows:

– **First Step**: Definition of defect type.
– **Second Step**: Decision between repairing/ regeneration [9].

- **Third Step**: Insertion of simultaneous implant placement or staged surgery.
- **Fourth Step**: Choice of regenerative technique.
- **Fifth Step**: Material of choice.

Techniques that best adapt to digital workflows are guided bone regeneration (GBR) and onlay block (OB) (Fig. 9.3).

9.2.4 Guided Bone Regeneration

GBR is based on the functional principle of the occlusive barrier by devices that prevent migration of epithelial cells to the site where colonization of osteo-progenitor elements is expected. Literature reports favorable results for the use of mechanical barriers that preserve a desired volume and prevent, as just said, epithelial cell migration. A physical graft is not necessarily needed to regenerate bone, as long as an area can be volumetrically stablished and protected by the means of a barrier.

According to some authors, for the success of this technique, the use of non-absorbable membrane is mandatory while others propose the use of absorbable membranes to reduce patient morbidity. Nevertheless, given its poor mechanical strength, these latest membranes require mechanical support to preserve the desired shape of the new bone gain.

Literature also agrees in the possibility of implant insertion simultaneous to GBR. Usually, although not biologically necessary, space maintenance is associated with biomaterials, used to fill the volume to be regenerated. This functional concept is based on the creation of a bone-driver site for blood colonization and future bone apposition, once isolated from the invasion of epithelial progenitor elements.

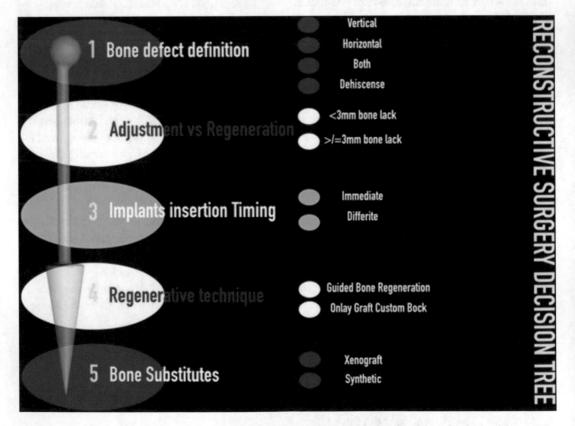

Fig. 9.3 Reconstructive bone surgery is a complex discipline. The image shows a decision tree based on techniques that, over the years, have proven to be the most suitable for each situation. Manual attitude of the operator is also considered

9.2.5 Onlay Grafting

This technique represents a valid alternative to GBR. Its regenerative principle is based on osteoconduction, functioning as a scaffold for subsequent invasion of newly synthesized bone tissue. Materials used can derive from autogenic, allogenic, xenogenic, or even synthetic origins. Depending on this, the block can also contain osteoinductive properties.

Conventional technique involves shaping and adapting the block to the recipient zone. Fixation and immobilization is fundamental. Covering membranes, usually absorbable ones, can be used.

Hydrolytic capacity of the material, and therefore its permeability, will depend on its macroscopic characteristics (texture). The more these characteristics meet vascular neoformation

requirements, the better and more efficient integration is achieved [9].

9.3 Digital Techniques

Digital techniques are extremely useful for reconstructive bone surgery. First of all, enhanced visualization allows bone deficiency to be framed very precisely, both in architectural and quantitative terms. In addition, CAD software eases design of any type of device used in surgery (Fig. 9.4). Production (CAM) also marks a revolution in terms of speed, costs, and working precision.

Starting from the assumption imposed by modern prosthetic concept, workflow digitalization makes possible to contextualize, and therefore harmonize, prosthetic restoration, implant and surrounding tissues (Figs. 9.5 and 9.6).

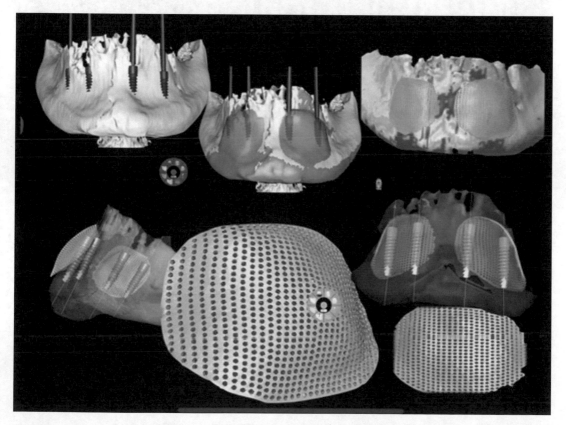

Fig. 9.4 In this sequence, a complete digital path is highlighted. Starting from data acquisition to accomplish custom mesh design for GBR surgery

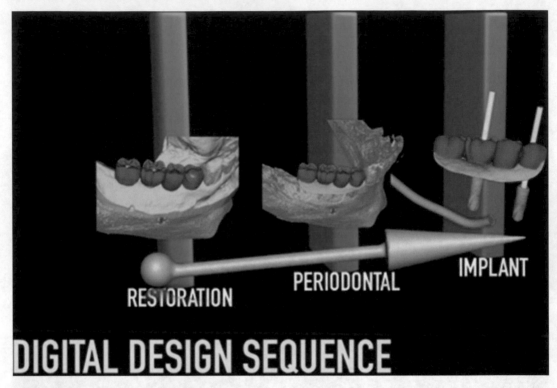

Fig. 9.5 Whether it is the acquisition of diagnostic data at check-in or the design phase, focus should always be put on relevant information regarding prosthetic restoration since this is the basis of any rehabilitation project. With this approach, it will be also easier to highlight a visualization of treatment objectives (VTO) in terms of implant-prosthetic aesthetics

9.3.1 Digital Workflow Concept

The expression "digital workflow," to date, is perhaps one of the mostly used in the academic-scientific world, as a promoter of cultural events and technical training. This phrase means the use of devices and software for the approach of clinical cases (Fig. 9.7). So, the workflow is actually a set of many technical and decision-making processes. It also distorts traditional information flow between clinician and laboratory, as some actions that were previously of strictly lab relevance have passed into the hands of the clinician, who is now becoming an active part of the design process.

9.3.2 Digital Reconstructive Surgery Concept

The term "digital approach to regenerative surgery" stands for a series of actions used to identify an alveolar tissue deficiency and plan its reconstructive phase, always in the context of an implant-supported prosthetic rehabilitation. The common denominator remains the planning of a reconstructive surgical phase from initial periodontal conditions, patient prosthetic requests and related needs in terms of implant support.

9.3.3 CAI Stage

The acquisition of clinical data consists of widely documented protocols, reported and disseminated scientifically. Said digital reconstructive surgical project should be strongly committed to complete functional rehabilitation of the masticatory system, regardless the extension of the sector to be rehabilitated. Therefore, the following recommendations can be drawn:

– DENTAL ARCHES. It is vital that registration of dental arches includes complete upper and lower jaws.

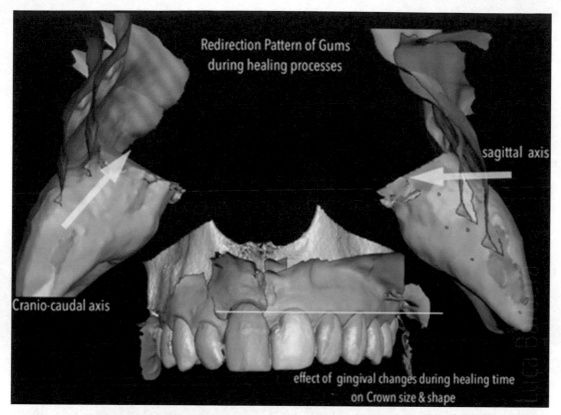

Fig. 9.6 Case of a patient with programmed extraction of tooth #11. Digital methods allow to predict results of soft tissue unfavorable healing following bone resorption. This helps clinicians plan a sequence of actions aimed to prevent bone resorption and compensate apical displacement of the gingival margin

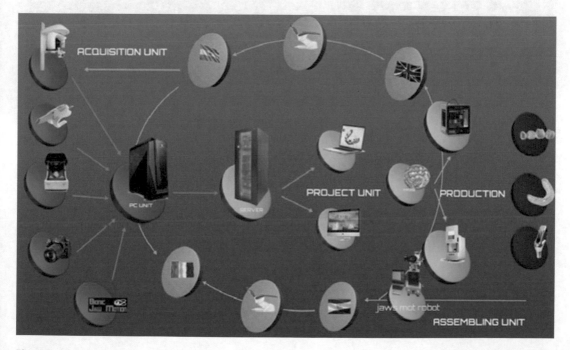

Fig. 9.7 Digital procedures summary

– SOFT TISSUES: Information on soft tissues is of vital importance for the evaluation of restoration and implant dimensions, emergence profile, and health prognosis. Moreover, they serve as indicators of the need of conducting regenerative projects.
– ALVEOLAR BONE SUPPORT. In general, information on hard tissues (alveolar bone support and teeth) is obtained through CBCT scans. They are difficult to obtain with an adequate level of quality due to artifacts that can "contaminate" sharpness of the returned images. Thus, emphasis must be put in collecting potentially combinable information to allow matching of the three main structures: teeth, gingiva/mucosa, and bone structures. In this way, the matching process will provide usable information for diagnostic visualization and design (See Chap. 1) (Figs. 9.8 and 9.9).

9.3.4 CAD Stage

The design of reconstructive surgery goes through some phases that alternate between prosthetic and surgical CAD software programs. As mentioned above, no regenerative or reconstructive design is carried out without a prosthetic project and the related implant support (Fig. 9.10).

Moreover, final evaluation on the type of reconstruction to be performed is carried out with virtual implant in situ and trying to avoid angled abutments as far as possible. Once said preset has been prepared, bone reconstruction design can take place. Depending on the needs, tissue augmentations will be designed to draw, on top of them, custom scaffolds to be fixed with screws or plates. Main phases of said design are described:

9.3.4.1 Step 1 Virtual Model
First phase involves construction of a three-dimensional virtual bone model from CBCT rendering (See Sect. 1.3.3, Chap. 1). This model must contain all information necessary for the subsequent design phase. Thus, depending on specific needs, different virtual models are created from CBCT and from surface scans by superimposing those images. In general, the following are evaluated: occlusion arches; opening arches (corresponding to CBCT position); soft gingival tissues; maxillary bones; prosthetic devices (Figs. 9.11 and 9.12).

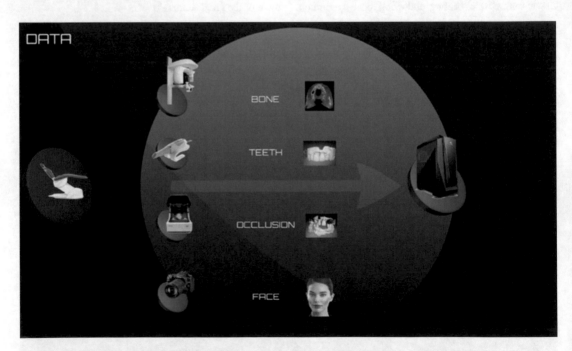

Fig. 9.8 Diagram illustrating digital acquisition methods of clinical data and relative instruments used for that means

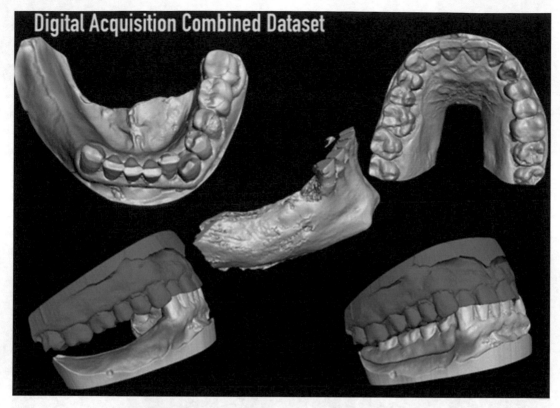

Fig. 9.9 Information needed should relate dental arches, soft tissues (gingiva and mucosa), occlusion, bone and additional patient prosthetic reference at the time of check-in, whenever possible

9.3.4.2 Step 2 Visualization of Treatment Objectives (VTO)

It starts from a problem list compilation derived from prosthetic, gingival and bone assessment to define vertical and horizontal concerns. A prosthetic-implant unit is designed and bone support availability is evaluated. At this point, a very precise idea about hard and soft tissue deficiencies can be assessed and therefore, the need for reconstructive surgery (Fig. 9.13).

9.3.4.3 Step 3 Project

The reconstructive surgical VTO is performed on a rendering containing alveolar bone support and definitive implant position. In this way, the assessment includes: type of bone deficiency related to implant ideal position (quality and quantity); reconstruction action deemed most suitable (reconstruction/regeneration); timing of implant placement (simultaneous/staged); regenerative technique (GBR/Onlay Block); material used (xenogenic/allo-

genic). Once this is done, a preliminary project of the necessary reconstructive step will be performed (as previously done for prosthetic-implant rehabilitation). On this later project, corresponding changes of the soft tissues will be evaluated (Fig. 9.14).

9.3.4.4 Step 4 Periodontal Approach

There is no reconstructive bone surgery project that does not also include a finalization step regarding periodontal soft tissues. In fact, every action that changes bone support architecture corresponds to soft tissue adaptation. Mucoperiosteal flaps are always coronally displaced following additive bone procedures, regardless of the technique or material chosen.

9.3.4.5 Step 5 Definitive Design

The design differs depending on whether a GBR or an OB technique is indicated. In the first case (GBR), the desired increase will be "drawn" over a duplicated virtual model of the sector of interest.

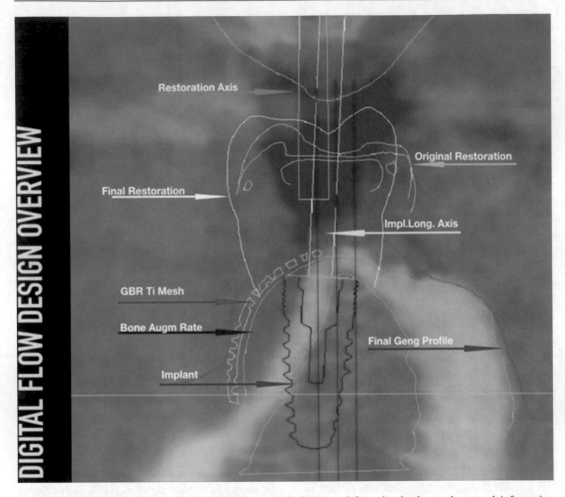

Fig. 9.10 All data obtained from digital design are automatically merged. It can be clearly seen how much information relating to the case study can be obtained and analyzed

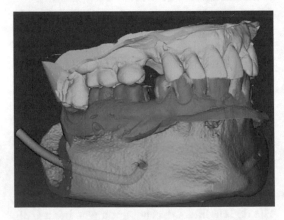

Fig. 9.11 Example of rendering ready for design of an implant-prosthetic rehabilitation in the lower arch

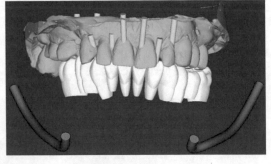

Fig. 9.12 Visualization of treatment objectives (VTO) as initial point to start for correct implant positioning and evaluation of any bone reconstructive surgery strategy

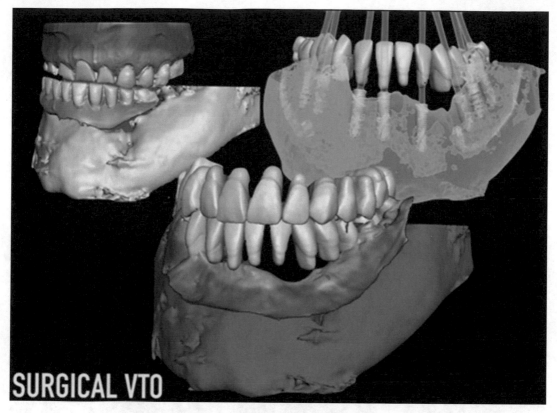

SURGICAL VTO

Fig. 9.13 Surgical VTO helps contextualize bone and gingival reconstruction necessary to obtain functional and aesthetically acceptable results

Then, a mesh is delimited using a rigid boxing system and determining thickness, texture, and offset characteristics. This project can be exported and sent directly to production sector. CAM process usually consists on sintering titanium material from powder, using a collimated laser beam (See Sect. 3.3.1.5, Chap. 3) [10]. In case of an OB technique, the design phase is more complex, as missing bone segment has to be created from a boolean subtraction action. That is, necessary bone augmentation is drawn over a copy of the maxillary bone model and then original bone model anatomy is subtracted by CAD means [11]. Additionally, if immediate implant insertion is foreseen, it is possible to create the implant bed directly into the molded block. Thus, surgical steps can be reduced (Figs. 9.15, 9.16 and 9.17).

9.3.5   CAM and Clinical Stages

Production technology of devices for reconstructive surgery is basically based on both printing and milling procedures. Blocks are milled from xenoplastic or synthetic materials. As for the containment devices used in GBR techniques, sintered titanium is mostly used and this is materialized by SLS 3D printing methods.

The clinical phase becomes less complex using these procedures, as it only involves exposing the surgical area and assembling materials already built. Titanium meshes and custom scaffolds should be always protected with membranes with extended barrier time characteristics and suturing should provide tension-free closure.

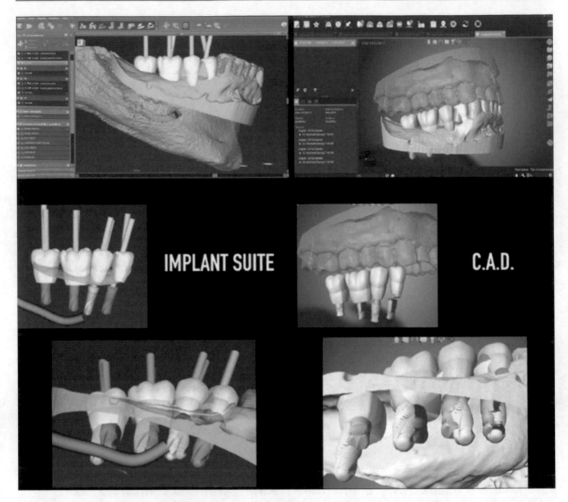

Fig. 9.14 Software for virtual implant placement and conventional CAD programs for the design of GBR and OB devices, interacting with each other in real time

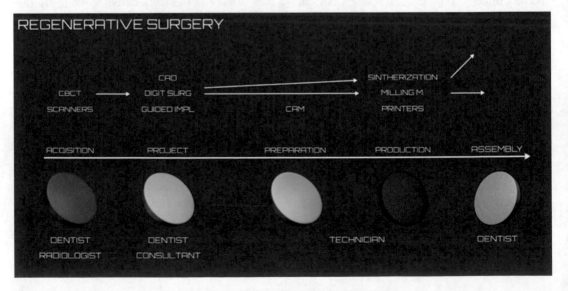

Fig. 9.15 Summary of steps used in digital design of reconstructive bone surgery

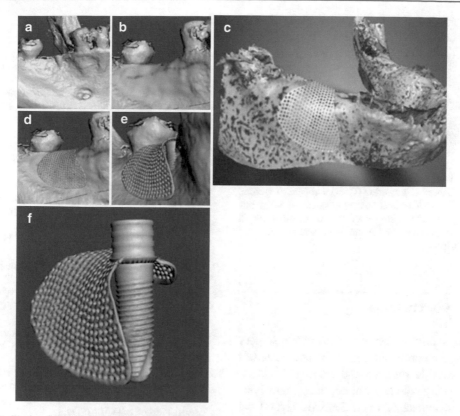

Fig. 9.16 Design flow of a titanium mesh for GBR. Evidence of implant dehiscence (**a**); virtual horizontal regeneration (**b**); CAD drawing of the titanium mesh (**c**); mesh visualization and relation to implant and anatomic structures (**d–f**)

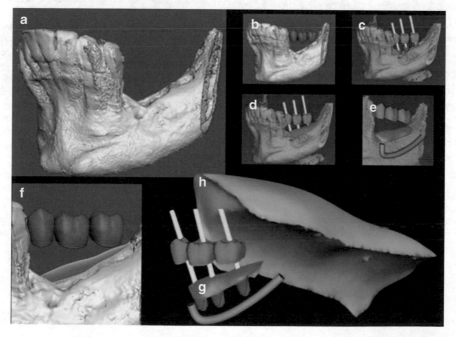

Fig. 9.17 Design flow of an Onlay Block (OB) for a case with severe vertical bone loss in the jaw. Bone area at check-in (**a**); prosthetic and implant VTO (**b**, **c**); surgical VTO with onlay and implants in position (**d**); global project rendering (**e–h**)

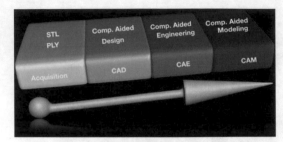

Fig. 9.18 Future of virtual design for prosthetic-surgical rehabilitations will be characterized by the use of Computer Aided Engineering (CAE) software programs, which will provide functional assessment of what has been designed. For example, assessment of block blood invasion in relation to fluid dynamics or even its resistance to implant load

9.4 Conclusions

Ongoing sophistication of reconstructive surgery schemes and continuous search for new materials require reliable research and functional evaluations. Healing outcome will depend on how bone defect and biomaterials are colonized by blood clot to allow vascular neoformation. Overall process described relies on osteoconductive characteristics. In the future, biomedical engineers should be included in the dental team to provide detailed information about biomechanics applied to regenerated tissues and its rehabilitation (Fig. 9.18).

CAD technology was born in the 1960s and ever since has been developing and finding applications in the most unimaginable technological fields. So today, as clinicians are able to experiment with biomaterials obtained by CAD-CAM procedures, dental community must consider itself ready to believe, foment and imagine new technical frontiers.

Bibliography

1. Klokkevold PR. Current status of dental implant: a periodontal perspective, vol. 15. Chicago: Quintessence Publishing; 2000. p. 1.
2. Le B, et al. Esthetic implant site development. Oral Maxillofac Surg Clin N Am. 2015;27:283–311.
3. Sonick M, Wang D. Implant site development. London: Wiley & Balckwell; 2012.
4. Deeb GR. Soft tissues grafting around teeth and implants. Oral Maxillofac Surg Clin N Am. 2015;27:425–48.
5. Yang Y. Evaluation and new classification of alveolar bone dehiscenses using cone beam computed tomography in vivo. Int J Morphol. 2015;33(1):361–8.
6. Chandra B. Periodonteal osseus defect: a review. CODS J Dent. 2017;9(1):22–29. https://doi.org/10.5005/jp-journals-10063-0028
7. Kumar P. Bone graft in dentistry. J Pharm Bioallied Sci. 2013;5(Suppl 1):S125–7.
8. Horowitz RA, et al. Bone grafting: history, rationale and selection of materials and techniques. Compend Contin Educ Dent. 2014;35:1–6.
9. Jaser RA. An overview of bone augmentation techniques. Clin Case Rep Rev. 2016;2(4):393–8. https://doi.org/10.15761/CCRR.1000226.
10. Sagheb K. Clinical outcome of alveolar ridge augmentation with individualized cad-cam produced titanium mesh. Int J Implant Dent. 2017;3:36. https://doi.org/10.1186/s40729-017-0097-z.
11. Gargiola U. Computer aided design/computer aided manufacturing of hydroxyapatite scaffold for bone reconstruction in jawbone atrophy: a systematic review and case report. Maxillofac Plast Reconstr Surg. 2016;38:5–9.
12. Liu J. Mechanism of guided bone regeneration: a review. Open Dent J. 2014;8(Suppl 1-M3):56–65.
13. Saad M. Guided bone regeneration: evidence and limits. Smile Dent J. 2012;7(1):8–16.
14. Yu N. Personalized scaffolding technologies for alveolar bone regenerative medicine. Orthod Craniofac Res. 2019;22(Suppl 1):69–75.
15. Rakhmatia YD. Current barrier membrane: titanium mesh and other membrane for guided bone regeneration in dental application. Ireland: Japan Prosthodontic Society. Elsevier; 2013.

Part IV

Guided Maxillofacial Surgery

3D Virtual Planning in Orthognathic Surgery

10

Eduardo D. Rubio, Gisela L. Nanni, and C. Mariano Mombrú

10.1 Introduction

Since the authors started working in the orthognathic surgery field, back in 1983, an obsession with the fact of achieving an accurate surgical planning arose. This meant a coincidence between planned results and those obtained.

Before digital photography era, the only way to obtain an approximate treatment result image was to calibrate photographs of patients to real size and make cuts and stickers on them in order to simulate the desired change. Getting photograph calibration was a difficult thing to do, because the person who developed the photo had to put a carbon copy on patient profile and enlarge the photo to match them. All that process was complicated and hence, not accurate enough (Fig. 10.1). The main concern at that time was to be sure that virtual planning was correct regarding soft tissue changes and bone movements, with an accurate mean ratio relationship [1]

At that time, one option was to do cephalometric tracing directly over the screen, in order to achieve greater precision when placing cephalometric points. Another option was doing it manually and then scanning it. Thereby, over the years, several methods were developed with the purpose of getting an accurate final image of the patient. Although several studies validated this new method, many orthodontists and surgeons decided to continue with traditional manual planning, as they were not convinced of its accuracy [1, 2].

E. D. Rubio (✉) · C. M. Mombrú
Oral and Maxillofacial Surgery Residency Program, School of Medical Sciences, Catholic University of Argentina, Buenos Aires, Argentina

Department of Oral and Maxillofacial Surgery, School of Dentistry, University of Buenos Aires, Buenos Aires, Argentina
e-mail: erubio@consultoriosrubio.com.ar

G. L. Nanni
Department of Oral and Maxillofacial Surgery, School of Dentistry, University of Buenos Aires, Buenos Aires, Argentina

Orthodontics Program, School of Dentistry, Del Salvador University, Buenos Aires, Argentina

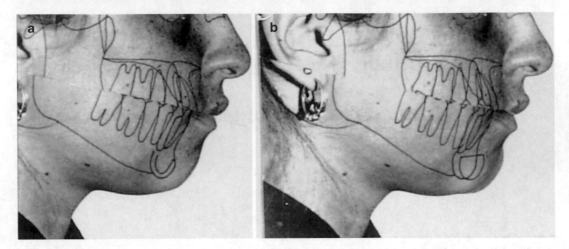

Fig. 10.1 (**a, b**) Carbon copy on patient profile with traditional manual planning

At first, the development of computed tomography (CT) improved bone pathology and maxillofacial trauma diagnosis, making a substantial progress on surgical planning. Later on, cone beam computed tomography (CBCT) emerged as a new tool, offering less radiation exposure compared with CT scans. Moreover, CBCT facilitated cortical thickness assessment in orthodontic planning, aiding treatment planning of arch expansion cases. In oral and maxillofacial surgery, this new technology had great impact, changing the entire surgical practice.

10.2 3D Virtual Planning

Main advantage of the digital era seems to be the ability to have patient information in a computer. Photos and dental casts merge with the CT providing three-dimensional and real size information. Thus, treatment planning is personalized according to each patient.

10.2.1 "Think more, less mistakes" Concept

Diagnostic imaging technology such as CT scanning, CBCT, and magnetic resonance imaging (MRI) have changed medical and dental practice. Similarly, dental software, surface scanners, and rapid prototyping machines had contributed to this digital revolution. This technology helps clinician explore patients thoroughly, from the smallest anatomical landmark to skin or tooth color, thanks to the brand-new 3D facial scanners.

Nowadays, there are many specialized laboratories responsible for processing images, printing models and guides with high precision and in a short period of time. Nevertheless, it is worth to mention that, as a surgeon, it is mandatory to understand the digital workflow. This is mainly to comprehend what study should be prescribed for each treatment in order to get an accurate outcome.

The use of traditional 2D orthognathic workup is associated with error and inaccuracies [2]. Many of these problems can be avoided with 3D virtual planning. Azarmehr et al. [3] summarized orthognathic 3D virtual planning literature, remarking its accuracy and efficiency in preoperative planning, whenever compared with conventional model surgery, and highlighting that surgical errors can be significantly decreased. Furthermore, a systematic review by Van den Bempt et al. [4] bassed on 16 studies, highlighted that 3D surgical cutting guides allowed accurate positioning of the maxillomandibular complex, according to the 3D virtual plan, in all directions.

Additionally, 3D virtual planning adds the benefit of time. Literature reports that the average preparation time for 3D planning is clearly reduced when compared to traditional orthognathic surgery planning [3]. Although digital planning can take more time prior to treatment (at least at the beginning), treatment tends to be more accurate and goals more precise and reliable. Therefore, think more during 3D virtual planning, less mistakes during surgery should be clinicians philosophy.

10.2.2   Data Acquisition (CAI)

10.2.2.1   The Patient

Patient clinical aspects are considered above all, whether the patient had finished his/her orthodontic treatment, or if it is a *surgery first consultation*. This means that clinical aspects outweigh cephalometric analysis, being critical during the decision-making process. Therefore, according to Arnett et al. [5] while cephalometric analysis indicates where the problem is, clinical aspects indicate how to solve it.

10.2.2.2   Facial Photos and 3D Scan

For an appropriate facial analysis, the *step- by-step process* described by Arnett and Gunson [6] and by Cifuentes et al. [7] is suggested. Once the patient leaves the office, facial photos previously taken are transcendental, as they allow the surgeon to take measurements, observe clinical aspects more precisely and start figuring out which treatment option could be the best. Therefore, facial photographs should be done thoroughly. A white background with side lighting is used to achieve a clear and neat image, avoiding shadows, just like in a traditional photo study (Fig. 10.2).

Before facial photos are taken, two landmarks must be made on patient skin, both on the forehead and on the right profile. In these two places two points are marked, separated from each other by two centimeters (Fig. 10.2). This arbitrary distance is used just to avoid mistakes. In the temple region, landmarks should have vertical orientation, because of the convexity of the area. This two centimeters distance is used to calibrate the image, enabling the clinician to enlarge the photograph to a real size within the software. Thus, starting from images with real size, real measurements, such as midline deviation, can be made.

Three photos from the frontal view are taken. One with relaxed lips, another smiling and a last one to evaluate the occlusal cant (Fig. 10.3). Additionally, a photo with cheek retractors showing the bite is taken (Fig. 10.4). Afterwards, a photo of the right profile with natural head position (NHP) according to Lundström and Lundström [8] is taken (Fig. 10.5). Also, a photography from below the mandible can be helpful to evaluate asymmetries. Finally, inferior facial third, and intraoral dental occlusion photographs are necessary to complete the record of the patient (Figs. 10.6, 10.7, 10.8).

10.2.2.3   Dental Cast Models, Scanners, and CBCT

The presence of orthodontic devices always tends to create artifact in patient CT images. For that reason, it is necessary to neatly overlap the acquired images with the dental arcs. There are three possibilities in order to do that:

1. *Dental cast models and CBCT (CBCT double scan)*
   On CT scan appointment, patient is asked to bring its dental casts articulated with a wax bite, previously prepared in the office. Then, two CBCT are taken using a bite index: one to the patient and another to the models. The wax bite used for both scans has ceramic devices added in order to enhance overlapping between both CT images within the software. This method tends to be the less accurate (Fig. 10.9).

2. *Dental arch scanning (IOS)*
   The two dental arches of the patient are scanned directly from the oral cavity with an intraoral scanner and an STL file is obtained. Afterwards, this STL file is overlapped using teeth references on the CT images. It is always recommended to include 2 cm of buccal gingiva and palatal wrinkles during the scanning process. This is to facilitate the merging process and assess potential errors. The main advantage of this method is decreasing distortion, due to the lack of dental impressions (Fig. 10.10).

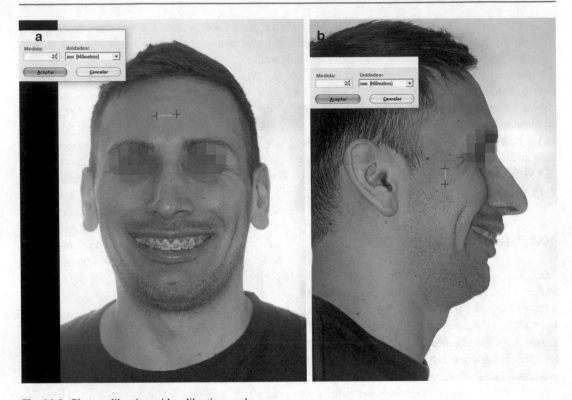

Fig. 10.2 Photo calibration with calibration marks

3. *Dental cast models scanning (EOS)*

Dental cast scanning is another method to achieve data acquisition (Fig. 10.11). In this case, an extraoral scanner is used to scan both jaws in the desire occlusion (treatment position). After that, the image obtained by the scan will be overlapped with the CT images (Fig. 10.12). This is one of the most sensitive steps, because an error at this point can result in an inaccurate splint. Whatever method used; software error should be, according to authors recommendation, less than 1 mm.

10.2.2.4 Imaging Modality

3D virtual planning has overridden 2D planning using lateral teleradiograph of the head. For 3D planning, CT is necessary. Selecting the appropriate imaging modality depends on spatial and contrast resolution. Spatial resolution is the ability for an image modality to differentiate two separate objects (i.e., a nerve canal within the mandible), whereas contrast resolution is the ability to differentiate image intensities between

two areas (i.e., fat stranding vs normal adipose tissue). Multislice tomography (MST) has high spatial resolution but is limited in contrast resolution. For this reason, MST is ideal for oral and maxillofacial cases because they often involve hard tissue interventions. Similarly, CBCT used in the appropriate surgical setting offers high spatial resolution with less radiation exposure, compared with MST. However, it has poor contrast resolution. [9, 10]

As mentioned in Chap. 1, field of view (FoV) of CBCT tomography equipments sometimes is not enough wide as required for the entire head of the patient (large FoV). Although this issue can be overcome by taking multiple scans with a smaller FoV and merging images within the software, precision could be jeopardized (Fig. 10.13).

Another drawback of this modality can could be its potential image distortion. Since it is not feasible to have a chin guard or bite device, patient must remain still during the study and slight movements can induce distortion of the final

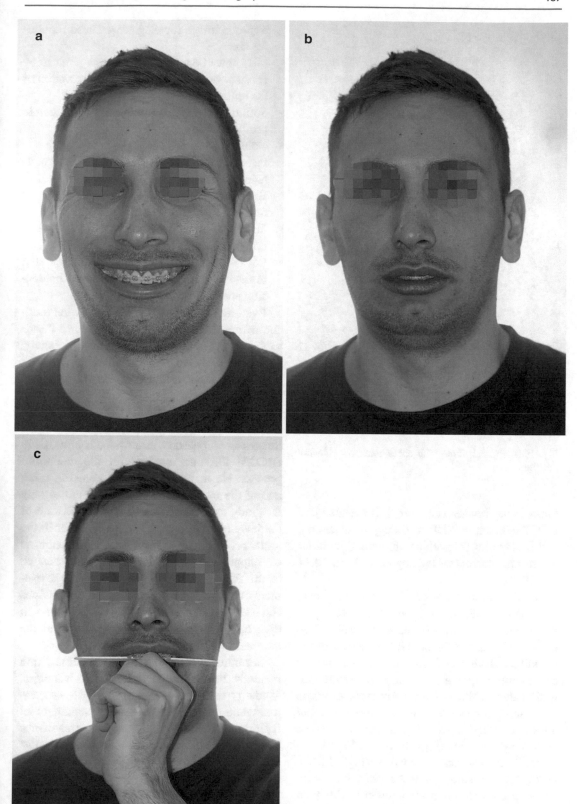

Fig. 10.3 (**a–c**) Extraoral frontal photos in NHP and occlusal cant evaluation

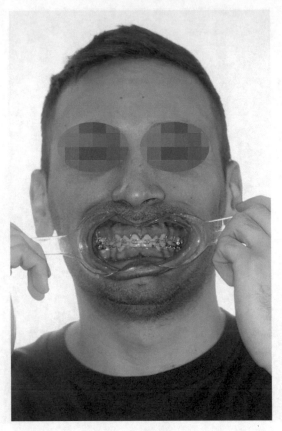

Fig. 10.4 Frontal photo with cheek retractors showing the bite

tomography image. Therefore, it is essential that CBCT is taken in NHP according to Lundström and Lundström [8] with no chin guard, in order to prevent blurring of the pogonion (Figs. 10.14 and 10.15).

In addition to the obstacles mentioned above, the image obtained with the CBCT often produces a blurring effect in the lateral wall of the maxillary sinus and in the third molar area of the mandible. Having an incomplete bone wall may cause complication at the moment of osteotomies design due to the lack of a flat surface. While this issue can be solved with a software tool that allows missing spaces filling, this process can be quite slow and tiring (Figs. 10.16 and 10.17).

MST is another alternative (Fig. 10.18). However, the study must be prescribed with some specific requirements in order to obtain an appropriate image for diagnosis. Those requirements are:

- MST must be taken from bregma point to 5th cervical vertebrae for adequate observation of the entire face.
- Soft tissue window is required for accurate profile analysis.
- No contrast agents are needed.
- Patient has to use the wax bite register for suitable jaw position during the scans.
- Eyes must be opened and lips must be resting.
- 3D reconstruction with 0.2 to 0.5 mm slice thickness should be prescribed as well.
- DICOM file exported into a CD is requested to the image laboratory and no slices impression are needed.

Even though this method is worldwide used, and with relative low cost, there are some disadvantages. If patient is not in NHP during the study, adjustments have to be made within the software to solve this issue. Additionally, working process tends to be slowed down due to the big number of image files provided with the CD.

Whether CBCT or MST is indicated, printed images are not needed, as described above. Only DICOM files are required for the diagnostic process. No matter what image modality used, one of the most important things is performing the study using a wax bite in centric relation of the jaw and with a gap of one millimeter in the molar area. The aim of this pitfall is to enhance overlapping between tomography and scanned teeth. Plus, wax bite avoids mandible movements during the study, and hence soft tissues can be analyzed in treatment position. Moreover, eyes being opened provide information at the moment of NHP.

In summary, regarding image modalities, both methods have advantages and disadvantages. Modality selection will depend on patient treatment requirements. CBCT is an outstanding tool for orthodontics and dental implant treatments. Conversely, MST could stand out as the most accurate method for orthognathic and reconstructive surgical planning, as NHP correction can be achieved within the software.

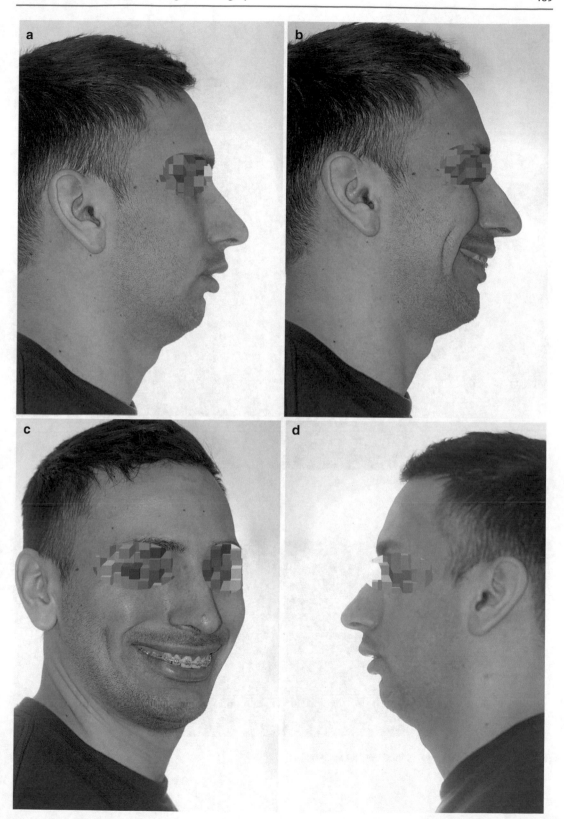

Fig. 10.5 (**a–f**) Extraoral photos in NHP. Right and left profiles

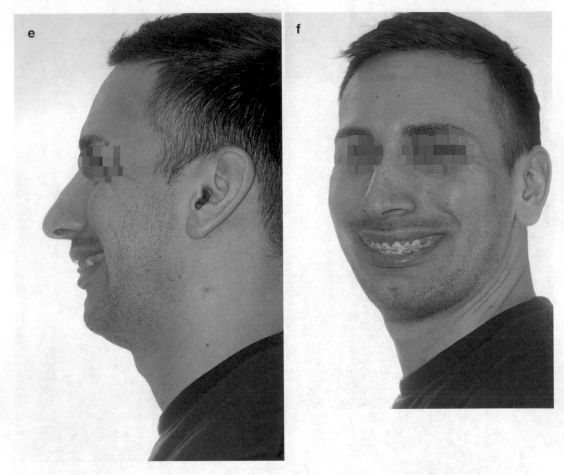

Fig. 10.5 (continued)

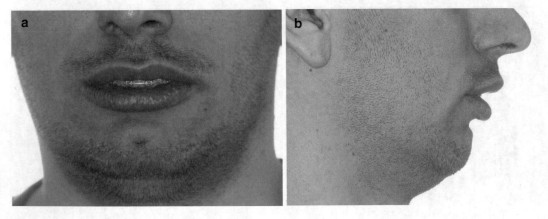

Fig. 10.6 (**a, b**) Inferior facial third clinical analysis

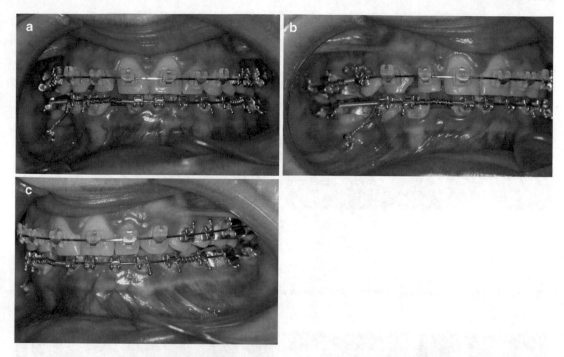

Fig. 10.7 (**a–c**) Class II patient intraoral photos

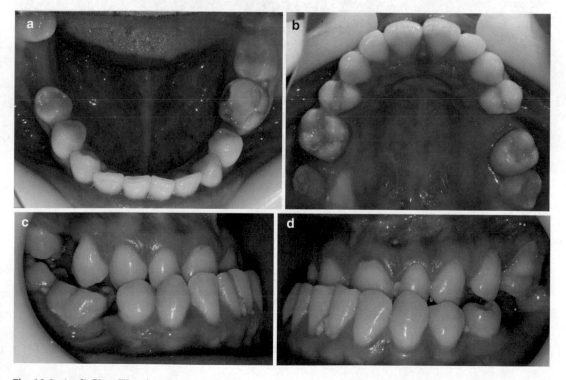

Fig. 10.8 (**a–d**) Class III patient intraoral photos

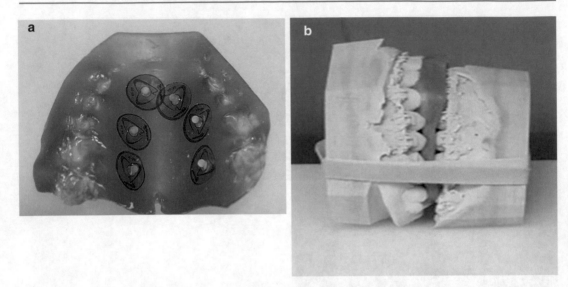

Fig. 10.9 (**a, b**) Dental cast models and wax bite register with ceramic devices for CBCT

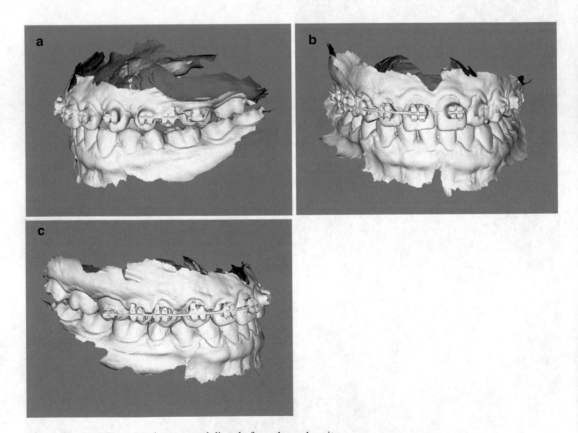

Fig. 10.10 (**a–c**) Dental arches scanned directly from the oral cavity

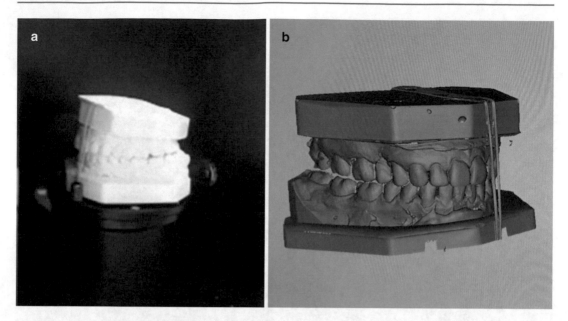

Fig. 10.11 (**a, b**) Dental cast model scanning

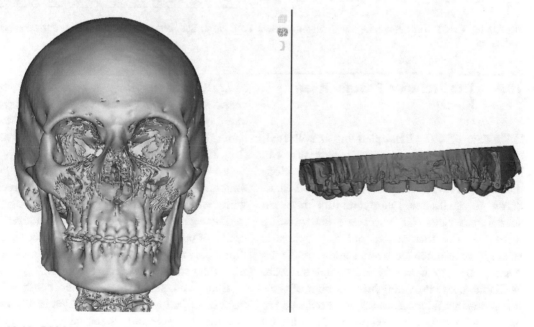

Fig. 10.12 DICOM and STL files merging process

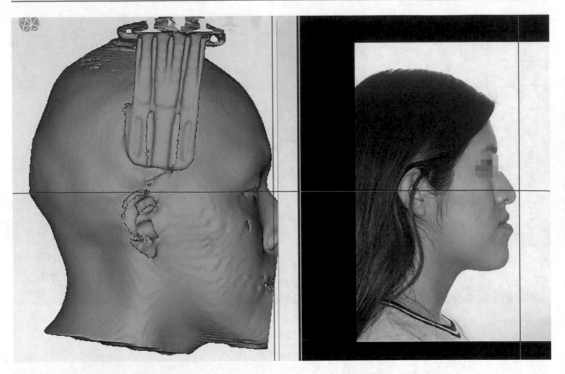

Fig. 10.13 CBCT soft tissue image with an insufficient FoV. Nose, lips, and chin are not visible for appropriate evaluation

10.3 The Planning Process Itself (CAD)

Once data for 3D virtual planning is collected, several dental and non-dental software can be used for planning. Open system development requires fulfilling of international standards to guarantee interoperability between scanning devices, CAD software and printing machines. For that reason, dental software is strongly recommended over a non-dental one. Among the great variety of dental software available, those providing high number of tools for patient variables assessment, should be the ones of choice (such as Nemofab Software by Nemotec®). Additionally, dental programs are usually designed by surgeons (i.e.: Dr. GW Arnett), according to patient surgical needs.

After NHP is achieved, cephalometric points are marked in the 3D cephalometric image. Those are: *nasion, basion, glabella, glabella Bl, subnasale, B point, pogonion, menton, cheek bone, subnasale, subpupil, frontozygomatic suture, mandibular angle, dental midlines, canine's cusps, upper and lower molars cusps* (Fig. 10.19).

Another option is to work with an orthopantomography, frontal and lateral teleradiographs, with the software, marking the points in the exact middle sagittal section (Fig. 10.20). Moreover, the option of being able to "surf" all CT slices brings thoroughly understanding of anatomic landmarks for a safer surgical procedure (Fig. 10.21).

Bone loss at the mandibular condyle has been described as a result of systemic and local arthritides, post-traumatic remodeling, hormonal imbalance and also, after orthognathic surgery. Therefore, temporomandibular joints (TMJ) must be evaluated before and throughout orthodontic–orthognathic treatment [11].

MRI has been considered the "gold standard" imaging tool to visualize disk position

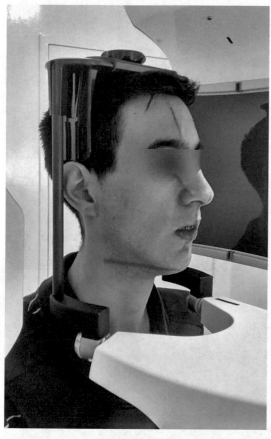

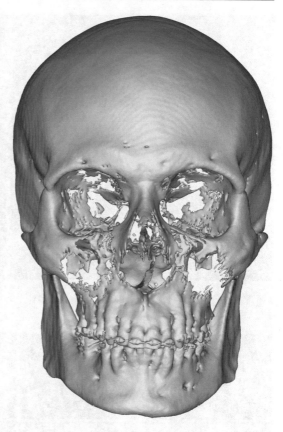

Fig. 10.16 Blurring effect of the maxillary sinus area

Fig. 10.14 No cephalostatic device needed for CBCT study

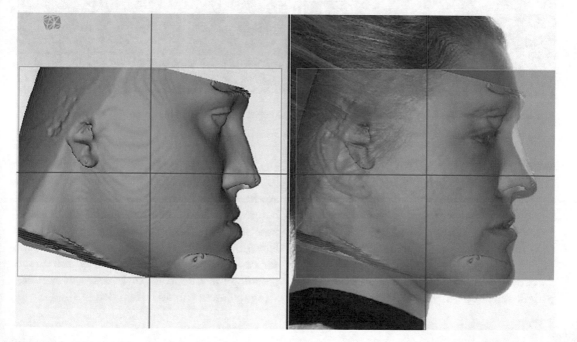

Fig. 10.15 Blurring of the chin area due to chin guard use

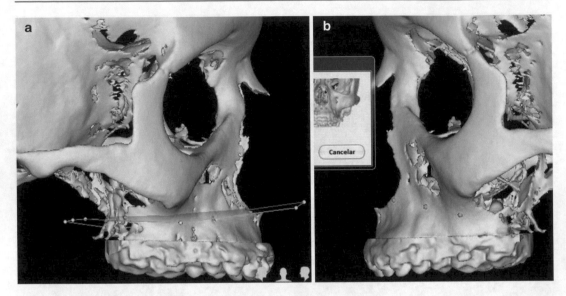

Fig. 10.17 (**a, b**) Osteotomies design in the maxilla

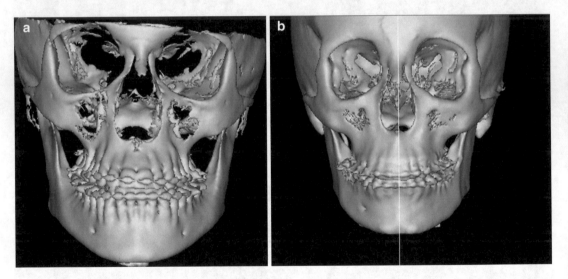

Fig. 10.18 (**a, b**) In MST, anterior wall of maxillary sinus structure has better definition, optimizing time

and to evaluate TMJ internal disk derangement [12]. This detailed evaluation of TMJ soft tissue structures is possible due to its superior contrast resolution when compared with CT scans [9]. Conversely, CBCT is considered the modality of choice for imaging the osseous components of the TMJ, due to its high spatial resolution and low radiation dose. Although no specific patient selection criteria has been published yet among literature regarding the use of CBCT for temporomandibular disorders, CBCT scans are needed to assess condyle cortical integrity before orthodontic and orthognathic treatment; especially in class II patients (Fig. 10.22). Nevertheless, MRI should precede CBCT for cases in which the diagnosis of soft tissue pathology is a concern, or in cases where ionizing radiation should be avoided [13].

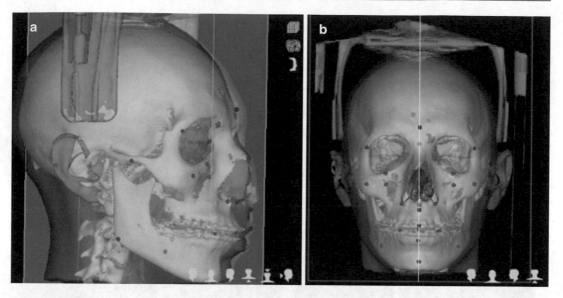

Fig. 10.19 (**a**, **b**) Lateral and frontal cephalometric points

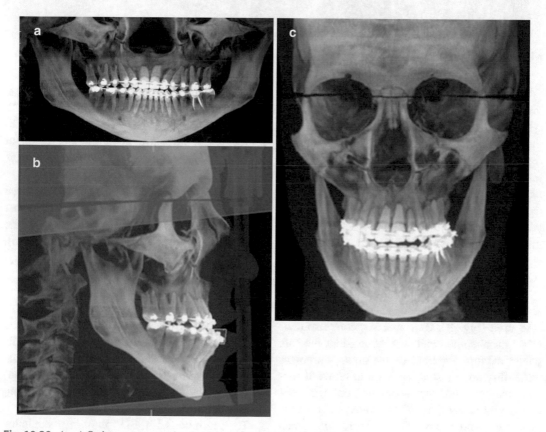

Fig. 10.20 (**a–c**) Orthopantomography, frontal and lateral teleradiographs

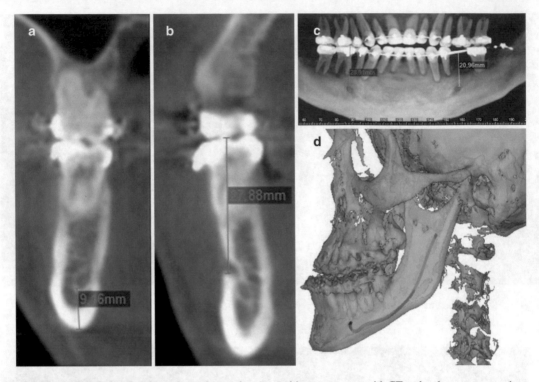

Fig. 10.21 (**a–d**) Inferior alveolar nerve and mental nerve position assessment with CT and orthopantomography

Another important tool whenever using CBCT images is volumetric quantification of the pharyngeal airway space (PAS) and, consequently, the localization of the narrowing or obstruction regions. This analysis has been incorporated into the diagnosis of orthodontic and orthognathic surgical planning, as obstructions or narrowing of the nasopharynx and/or oropharynx can be present in patients with an altered maxillo-mandibular relation and can be also related to obstructive sleep apnea syndrome (OSAS) [14].

Results of airway volume could be variable, since there are several ways to delimitate the PAS area (Fig. 10.23). Some surgeons use posterior nasal spine, while others consider the soft palate as superior limit of the area. Moreover, variability among study designs, in terms of surgical methods, imaging techniques, defined landmarks on radiographs, different uses of software programs, and many other factors, aggravates comparison and blurs the meaning of linear and

volumetric PAS measurement results. Therefore, uniform measure criterion of PAS using CBCT should be an important issue to solve, in order to achieve a reliable follow-up of surgical treatment for mandibular prognathism and in the diagnosis of OSAS [15].

However, regardless PAS boundaries considered for measurements, most of the studies claim that three-dimensional design of PAS seems to be the most reliable and precise measuring method [14, 15].

Next step in 3D virtual planning is to design osteotomies in the maxilla, the mandible and the chin, if needed. Regardless of the dentofacial anomaly diagnosis and treatment plan, a Le Fort I (LFI) osteotomy design is normally used in the maxilla, while both unilateral or bilateral sagittal split osteotomy (SSO) and/or intraoral vertical ramus osteotomy (IVRO) are used in the mandible. Finally, genioplasty is planned according to each case (Fig. 10.24).

To continue with 3D planning, cephalometric tracings is performed in the usual way

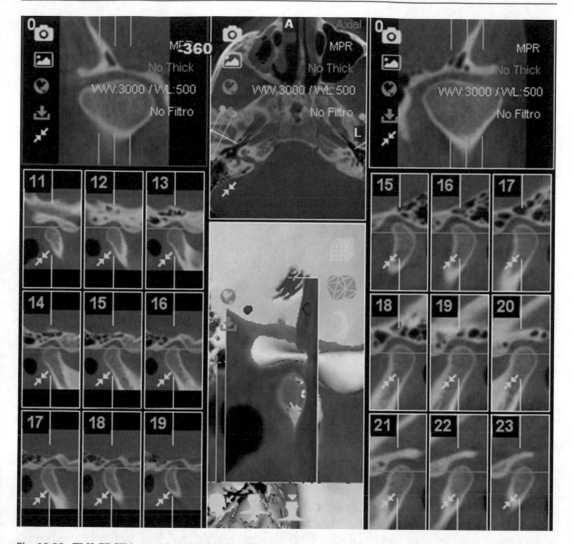

Fig. 10.22 TMJ CBCT images for condyle cortical integrity assessment

(Fig. 10.25). Although this "step-by-step" process is not so different than traditional planning, surgeons who use free movements tend to skip some of these steps. Software programs suggest which changes should be made to go forward with the planning in order to complete the movements in a three-dimensional way. According to that, middle dental line, palatine plane, pitch, roll, and yaw movements, among others, are manually marked for both jaw and chin (Fig. 10.26).

At this point, it is possible to consider all surgical movements in concordance with the orthodontic treatment plan and potential handling of several variables, until the desired result is achieved. Furthermore, a software tool provides a summary of all movements needed. Since bone contours are always irregular, possible bone interferences can be identified as well (Fig. 10.27d). Finally, software rebuilds the skin of the patient in order to assess whether the result of the planned surgery is adequate in relation to soft tissues (Fig. 10.27).

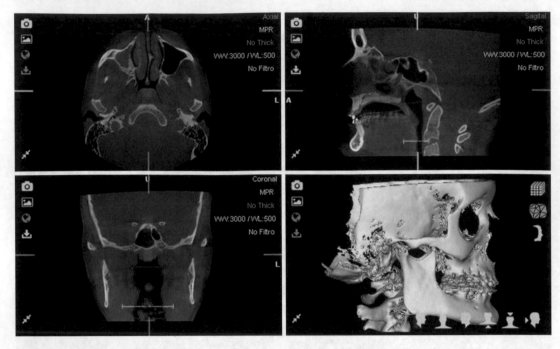

Fig. 10.23 Volumetric posterior airway space (PAS) analysis by CBCT images

10.4 3D Printing (CAM)

Once the entire creative planning process is completed, intermediate and final splints fabrication is carried out. Decision has to be made, whether the surgery will be a "mandible first surgery" or not; in order to define which jaw will be mobilized first. Afterwards, some dental points have to be traced according to the desired depth of the splint, to allow for proper fitting in the dental arch during surgery. If there is no space between dental arches, it is necessary to open the bite for some millimeters (Fig. 10.28).

Once the desired result is obtained, it is necessary to export the splint STL file so that a 3D printing can be made. General considerations about 3D printing methods and materials are described in Chap. 3.

The most used printing methods in maxillofacial surgery are: Fused Deposition Material (FDM) and stereolithography (SLA/DLP).

Among the 3D printing materials used in these cases for the FDM technique method, PLA (polyacetic acid) and ABS (Acrylonitrile butadiene styrene) are the most popular. On the other hand, biocompatible resins (those usually labeled as "Surgical Guide Resins") are needed for SLA and DLP methods. Additionally, these materials can tolerate steam sterilization processes and deliver final isotropic mechanical properties, compared to FDM materials. For those reasons and because of its accuracy, stereolithography is the best option for surgical guide printing.

10.5 Osteotomies Surgical Guides Making Process

Some of the greatest errors of 3D virtual planning come from modifications planned on the "Z axis" and vertical movements of the max-

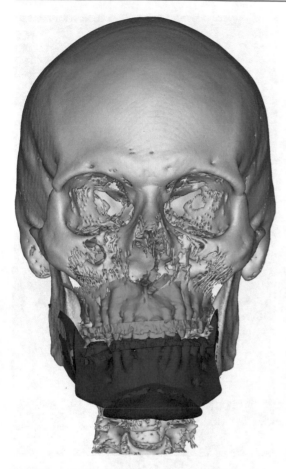

Fig. 10.24 Maxilla, mandible, and chin osteotomies design

illa, since neither the analog nor the digital splint transmit the planned movements in a vertical direction (impaction or down-graft movements).

Other common and significant error, which surgical splints cannot solve, are those regarding the condyle–fossa relation. The position of the maxilla depends on the mandibular position after its auto-rotational movement. Therefore, success depends on proper position of the condyles inside the glenoid fossa, resulting this in a potential problem at the moment of repositioning the maxilla during surgery. Thus, one of 3D virtual planning most important achievements is the possibility of treating each patient individually from their CT images.

Nowadays splint-less surgeries are also possible, thanks to CAD software and titanium printing machines (Fig. 10.29). In these protocols, the information of jaw new position is given by a bone-supported osteotomy guide and printed titanium plates (Fig. 10.30).

10.6   Other Indications and Limitations

3D virtual planning is a powerful tool with several indications, besides orthognathic surgery. A loose bone fragment after a sagittal split osteotomy, due to infection, can be an example of 3D planning indication (Fig. 10.31). Customized devices for bone fixation can also be used to obtain good mandibular contour, as well as proper union of the bone fragments (Fig. 10.32).

Besides orthognathic surgery, 3D virtual planning is also used for osteogenic distraction surgery, reconstructive surgery, and maxillofacial trauma. Additionally, computer planning is used for navigation during difficult 3D movement, in special cases and in complex reconstructive surgery [16].

3D planning is extensively used for maxillofacial pathology diagnosis, thanks to the possibility of virtually visualizing pathology and providing guidance for the location of resection margins. In some cases, where midface pathologies (such as tumors within the maxillary sinus or nasal cavity) require osteotomies without direct visualization, surgical planning allows for such resections to be performed with great confidence.

Moreover, according to literature, 3D guided surgery has been reported to be 60–120 minutes faster in microvascular tissue transfers using a bony donor site, such as the fibula osteocutaneous free flap, when compared to non-guided surgery [17].

In the setting of maxillofacial trauma, 3D planning allows fabrication of customized implants. Features of 3D planning in midface reconstruction, especially during orbital repair, help improve outcomes of complex maxillofacial trauma [9].

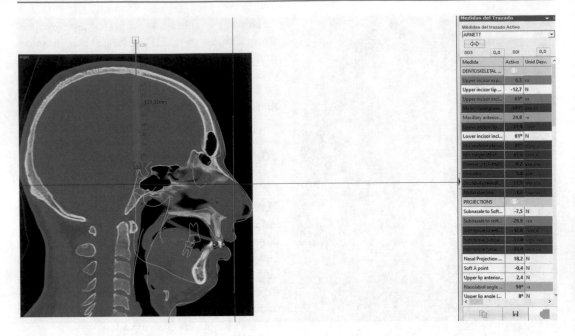

Fig. 10.25 Cephalometric tracing

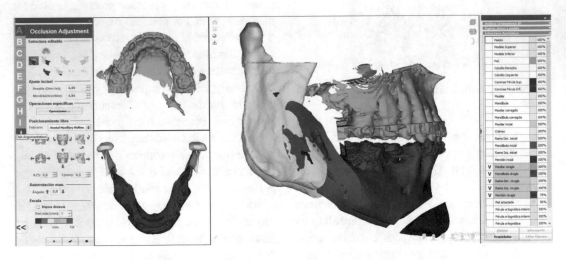

Fig. 10.26 Osteotomies and jaws movements

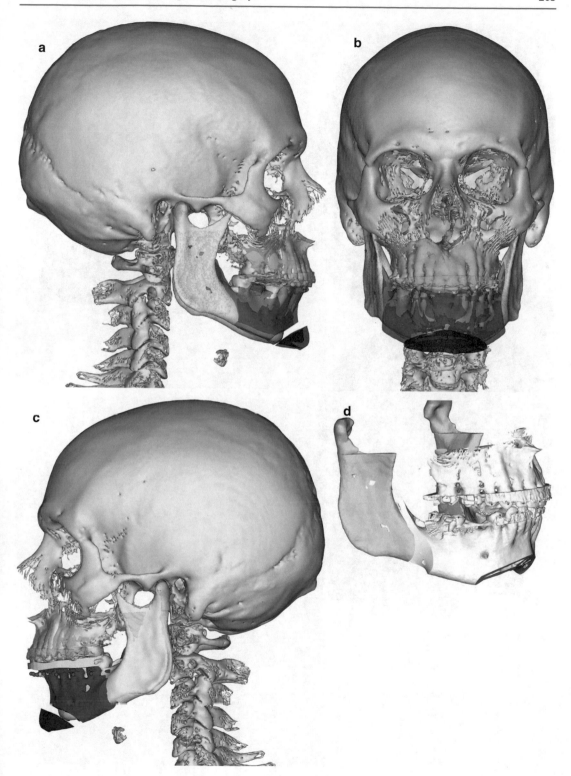

Fig. 10.27 (**a–c**) 3D frontal and lateral planning. (**d**) Bone interferences identification. (**e–g**) morphing process. (**h, i**) presurgical and postsurgical facial aspect

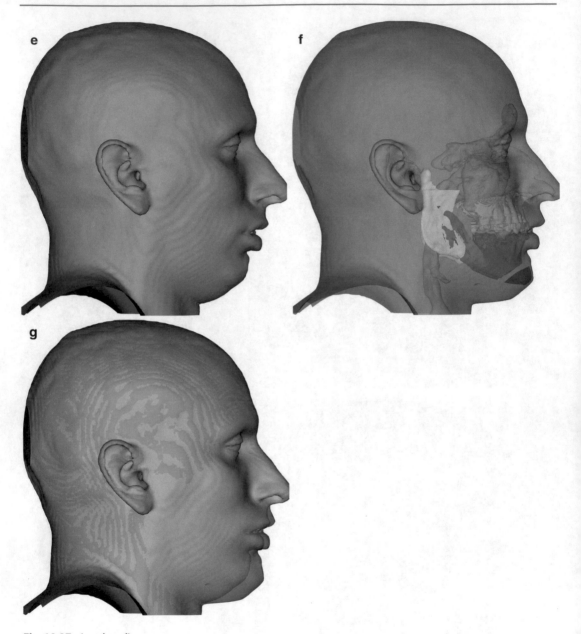

Fig. 10.27 (continued)

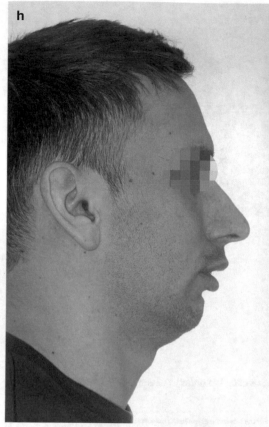
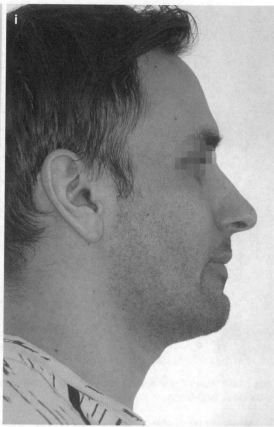

Fig. 10.27 (continued)

There are not known contraindications to 3D virtual planning. However, financial constraints may be a detrimental factor, as costs include hardware, software, and fees for processing the information, together with splint and models fabrication [18].

	Traditional planning	Virtual surgical planning
Scope	1 dimension	Volumetric, 3 dimensions, adds soft tissues
Patient information	Good	Excellent
Prediction accuracy	Good	Excellent

10.7   Conclusion

In summary, a small comparison between traditional and 3D virtual planning methods is presented:

	Traditional planning	Virtual surgical planning
Cost	Low	High
Learning curve	Short	Long
Precision	Enough	High

Technology faces us to an exciting world, which continues to evolve day by day.

Orwell's famous novel, titled "1984," written in 1949, stated that reality imitates art. In fact, the term "big brother", used nowadays, was mentioned at that time by the author. Moreover, genetic manipulation used in the film "Jurassic Park" seemed something made for movies only. However, nowadays defective mitochondria may be modified to treat some genetic diseases.

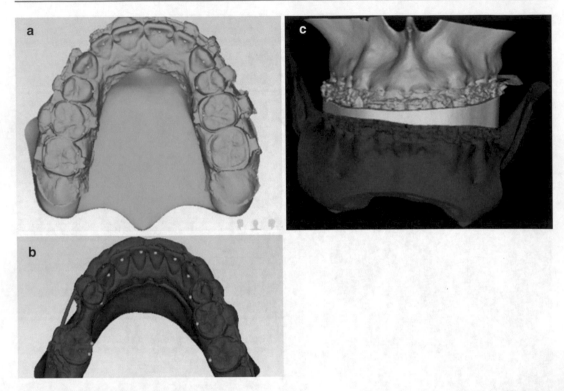

Fig. 10.28 (**a–c**) Splint printing process. Dental landmarks are traced in order to obtain a proper fitting guide for jaw position during surgery

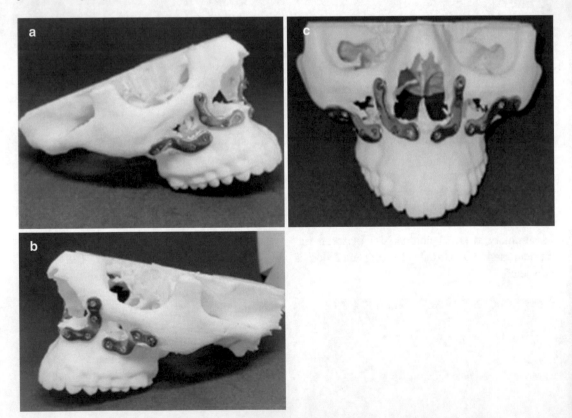

Fig. 10.29 (**a–c**) Customized titanium plates with the new 3D position in the stereolithographic model

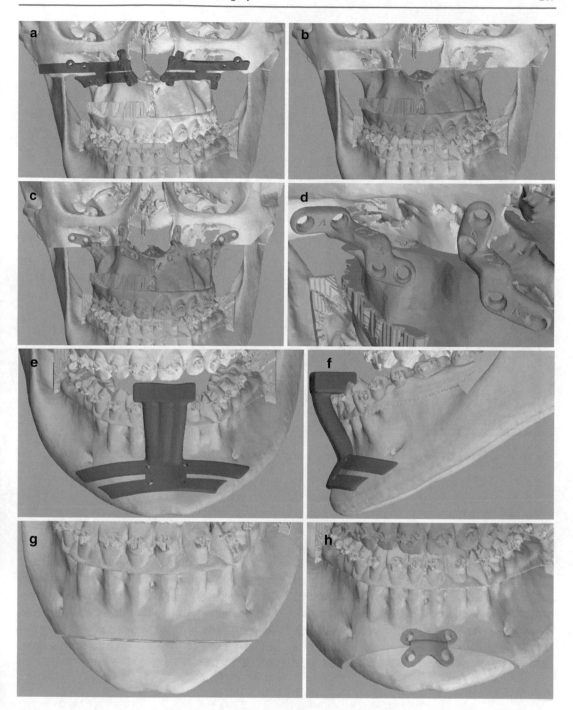

Fig. 10.30 (**a–h**) Splint-less and bone-supported guide surgery planning. Osteotomy guides are fixed to the bone to lead bone cuts. Each hole is designed to fit both guide and customized titanium plates

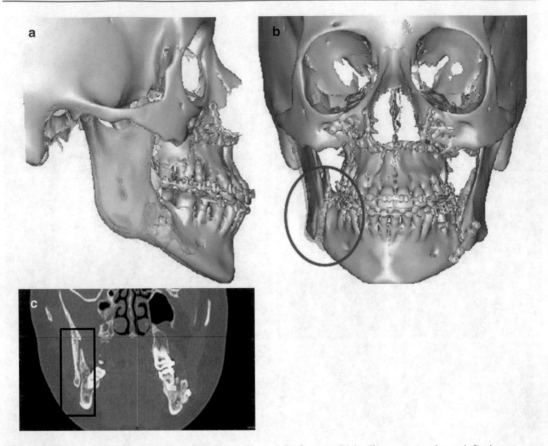

Fig. 10.31 (**a–c**) CBCT image showing loose bone fragments after a sagittal split osteotomy due to infection

Those who have made splints manually in the past, and do them digitally now, can judge consistently what this advance means. It can be said that clinicians are at the beginning of a diagnostic and industrial revolution, in terms of daily work in orthodontics and orthognathic surgery. The foundations described in this chapter attest to this. 3D virtual planning is here to stay, and already constitutes the gold standard to treat many cases, such as facial asymmetries.

Finally, 3D virtual planning will continue to improve during time, for sure, and methodology for patient data processing will evolve quickly. The authors hope to be witnesses of those changes, with the main purpose of providing better life quality to patients. Authors have no conflict of interest.

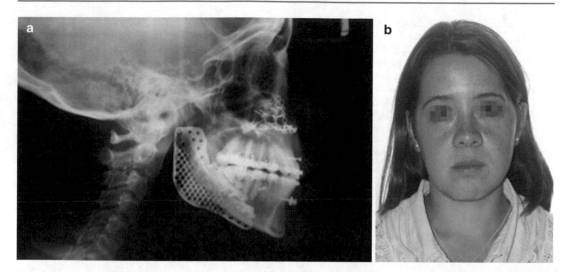

Fig. 10.32 (**a, b**) Bone fixation with customized devices for mandibular contour smoothness and proper union of bone fragments. Facial aspect after surgery

References

1. Rubio ED, Pascual AM, Garcia Casanova MC, Madrazo MJ. Predicción cefalométrica para cirugía ortognática. Ortodoncia. 2006;69(139):16–23.
2. Wang Y, Jingtao L, Yinglin X, Ning H, Jihua L. Accuracy of virtual surgical planning-assisted management for maxillary hypoplasia in adult patients with cleft lip and palate. J Plast Reconstr Aesthet Surg. 2020;73(1):134–40.
3. Azarmehr I, Stokbro K, Bell RB, et al. Surgical navigation: a systematic review of indications, treatments, and outcomes in oral and maxillofacial surgery. J Oral Maxillofac Surg. 2017;75(9):1987–2005.
4. Van den Bempt M, Liebregts J, Maal T, et al. Toward a higher accuracy in orthognathic surgery by using intraoperative computer navigation, 3D surgical guides, and/or customized osteosynthesis plates: a systematic review. J Craniomaxillofac Surg. 2018;46(12):2108–19.
5. Arnett GW, Jelic JS, Kim J, Cummings DR, Beress A, Worley CM Jr, Chung B, Bergman R. Soft tissue cephalometric analysis: diagnosis and treatment planning of dentofacial deformity. Am J Orthod Dentofac Orthop. 1999;116(3):239–53.
6. Arnett GW, Gunson MJ. Facial planning for orthodontists and oral surgeons. Am J Orthod Dentofac Orthop. 2004;126(3):290–5.
7. Cifuentes J, Teuber C, Gantz A, Barrera A, Danesh G, Yanine N, Lippold C. Facial soft tissue response to maxillo-mandibular advancement in obstructive sleep apnea syndrome patients. Head Face Med. 2017;13(1):15.
8. Lundström F, Lundström A. Natural head position as a basis for cephalometric analysis. Am J Orthod Dentofac Orthop. 1992;101(3):244–7.
9. Hua J, Aziz S, Shum JW. Virtual surgical planning. Oral Maxillofac Surg Clin North Am. 2009;31(4):519–30.
10. Pauwels R, Beinsberger J, Stamatakis H, et al. Comparison of spatial and contrast resolution for cone beam computed tomography scanners. Oral Surg Oral Med Oral Pathol Oral Radiol. 2012;114(1):127–35.
11. Gunson MJ, Arnett GW, Milam SB. Pathophysiology and pharmacologic control of osseous mandibular condylar resorption. J Oral Maxillofac Surg. 2012;70(8):1918–34.
12. Al-Saleh MAQ, Alsufyani N, Lai H, Lagrave M, Jaremko JL, Major PW. Usefulness of MRI-CBCT image registration in the evaluation of temporomandibular joint internal derangement by novice examiners. Oral Surg Oral Med Oral Pathol Oral Radiol. 2017;123(2):249–56.
13. Alkhader M, Kuribayashi A, Ohbayashi N, Nakamura S, Kurabayashi T. Usefulness of cone beam computed tomography in temporomandibular joints with soft tissue pathology. Dentomaxillofac Radiol. 2010;39(6):343–8.
14. Torres HM, Evangelista K, Torres EM, Estrela C, Leite AF, Valladares-Neto J, Silva MAG. Reliability and validity of two software systems used to measure the pharyngeal airway space in three-dimensional analysis. Int J Oral Maxillofac Surg. 2020;49(5):602–13.
15. Burkhard JP, Dietrich AD, Jacobsen C, Roos M, Lübbers HT, Obwegeser JA. Cephalometric and three-dimensional assessment of the posterior airway space and imaging software reliability analysis before

and after orthognathic surgery. J Craniomaxillofac Surg. 2014;42(7):1428–36.

16. Swennen GJ, Mollemans W, De Clercq C. A cone-beam computed tomography triple scan procedure to obtain a three-dimensional augmented virtual skull model appropriate for orthognathic surgery planning. J Craniofac Surg. 2009;20(2):297–307.

17. Chang EI, Jenkins MP, Patel SA, et al. Long-term operative outcomes of preoperative computed tomog-raphy-guided virtual surgical planning for osteo-cutaneous free flap mandible reconstruction. Plast Reconstr Surg. 2016;137(2):619–23.

18. Drew SJ. Computer planning for orthognathic sur-gery. In: Kademani D, Tiwana P, editors. Atlas of oral & maxillofacial surgery. Part IV. Orthognathic and craniofacial surgery, vol. 28. St. Louis: Saunders, Elsevier; 2016. p. 263–81.

Printed in the United States
by Baker & Taylor Publisher Services